Understanding of Stroke Mechanisms

Based on the MRI/A Findings of Clinical Cases

Understanding of Stroke Mechanisms

Based on the MRI/A Findings of Clinical Cases

Printed in Seoul, Republic of Korea
ISBN 978-89-521-1251-4 (93510)

Seoul National University Press
1Gwanak-ro, Gwanak-gu, Seoul 151-742, Republic of Korea

E-mail: snubook@snu.ac.kr
Home-page: http://www.snupress.com
Tel: 82-2-880-5252
Fax: 82-2-889-0785
First Printing: Sep. 30, 2011
Second Printing: Aug. 31, 2012

2012 Excellent Books of Basic Sciences
(Selected by the National Academy of Sciences, Republic of Korea)

Understanding of Stroke Mechanisms

Based on the MRI/A Findings of Clinical Cases

Jae-Kyu Roh, M.D., Ph.D.

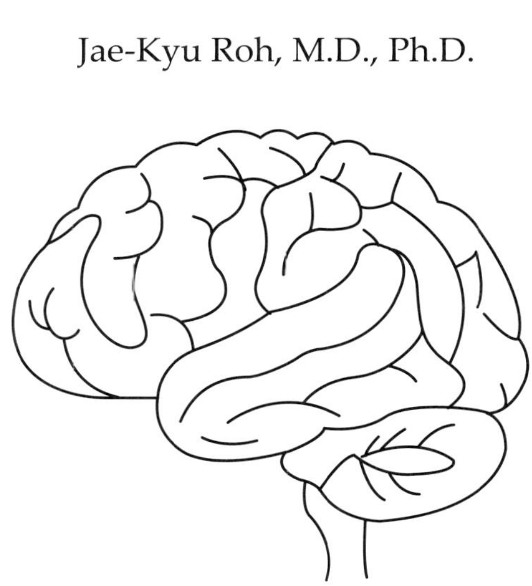

SNUPRESS
Seoul National University Press

PROLOGUE

The pathogenesis of stroke is various and is one of the most complicated among the diseases responsible for worldwide mortality and morbidity. The incidence of stroke increases dramatically with advancing age. A number of factors that can be classified as modifiable and unmodifiable increase the risk of ischemic stroke. Risk factors for ischemic stroke include old age, male gender, hypertension, diabetes mellitus, dyslipidemia, heart disease, smoking, excessive alcohol intake, obesity, and a family history of stroke. These risk factors directly or indirectly induce endothelial dysfunction, atherosclerosis, thrombosis, or embolization, contributing to the various phenotypes of ischemic stroke. These risk factors change with age and life style. The main mechanisms of stroke include large artery atherosclerosis, cardioembolism, and small vessel occlusion. Early identification of the underlying vascular mechanisms can prevent fatal complications and the progression or recurrence of stroke. Neuro-imaging characteristics differ according to the thrombo-embolic mechanisms, but non-specific manifestations frequently occur in inconsistent patterns. Moreover, two or more causes, or rare vascular pathologies often induce stroke, which makes it difficult to establish the patho-mechanism. The increasing availability of MRI and the advent of new imaging techniques, especially DWI and MRA, have helped us to better understand the mechanisms of stroke. But the first step in classifying the underlying mechanisms is the careful evaluation of the patient through history taking and the neurological examination. This case collection contains all the major aspects of typical, atypical, and combined mechanisms of stroke, primarily focusing on ischemic stroke. In this collection, each case is described with four items; clinical features, neuroimaging findings, clinical course, and comprehensive information on the putative mechanisms. In the last part, several interesting and instructive cases are described in terms of pathognomonic findings, therapeutic concerns, and recovery mechanisms. The stroke mechanism in this book is solely based on my personal decision and therefore, other stroke expert may have different opinions in some cases. This issue can be answered by forthcoming more sophisticated techniques such as plaque imaging, etc. This book is aimed at improving diagnostic skills of students, residents, and stroke physicians, by providing accurate knowledge regarding the mechanism of various stroke cases under general as well as specific situations. Further, this book offers a contemporary and authoritative view of acute and chronic care for stroke patients.

I would like to thank to doctors Kyoung-Bok Lee and Keun-Hwa Jung for their contribution to the collection of the cases and the final editing of this book. Finally, I would dedicate cordially this book to all my patients who have taught me through their illness.

CONTENTS

CASE SUMMARY

ID	Classification	Mechanism	Specific category
1	Large Artery Atherosclerosis	Artery to Artery Embolism	Aortic Arch Disease
2	Large Artery Atherosclerosis	Artery to Artery Embolism	Aortic Arch Disease
3	Large Artery Atherosclerosis	Artery to Artery Embolism	CCA Disease
4	Large Artery Atherosclerosis	Artery to Artery Embolism	Aortic Arch, pICA Disease
5	Large Artery Atherosclerosis	Artery to Artery Embolism	pICA Disease
6	Large Artery Atherosclerosis	Artery to Artery Embolism	pICA Disease
7	Large Artery Atherosclerosis	Artery to Artery Embolism	Bilateral Infarcts via Acom
8	Large Artery Atherosclerosis	Artery to Artery Embolism	dICA Disease
9	Large Artery Atherosclerosis	Artery to Artery Embolism	dICA Disease
10	Large Artery Atherosclerosis	Artery to Artery Embolism	dICA Disease
11	Large Artery Atherosclerosis	Artery to Artery Embolism	dICA Disease
12	Large Artery Atherosclerosis	Artery to Artery Embolism	dICA Disease
13	Large Artery Atherosclerosis	Artery to Artery Embolism	ICA Tandem Disease
14	Large Artery Atherosclerosis	Artery to Artery Embolism	pICA, MCA Disease
15	Large Artery Atherosclerosis	Artery to Artery Embolism	MCA Disease
16	Large Artery Atherosclerosis	Artery to Artery Embolism	MCA Disease
17	Large Artery Atherosclerosis	Artery to Artery Embolism	dMCA Disease
18	Large Artery Atherosclerosis	Artery to Artery Embolism	ACA Disease
19	Large Artery Atherosclerosis	Artery to Artery Embolism	ACA Disease
20	Large Artery Atherosclerosis	Artery to Artery Embolism	VA orifice Disease
21	Large Artery Atherosclerosis	Artery to Artery Embolism	VA Disease
22	Large Artery Atherosclerosis	Artery to Artery Embolism	VA Disease
23	Large Artery Atherosclerosis	Artery to Artery Embolism	VA Disease
24	Large Artery Atherosclerosis	Artery to Artery Embolism	VA Disease
25	Large Artery Atherosclerosis	Artery to Artery Embolism	VA, BA Disease
26	Large artery atherosclerosis	Artery to artery embolism	VA, BA Disease
27	Large Artery Atherosclerosis	Artery to Artery Embolism	BA Disease
28	Large Artery Atherosclerosis	Artery to Artery Embolism	Amaurosis Fugax
29	Large Artery Atherosclerosis	Artery to Artery Embolism	Amaurosis Fugax
30	Large Artery Atherosclerosis	In Situ Thrombosis	MCA Disease
31	Large Artery Atherosclerosis	In Situ Thrombosis	MCA Disease
32	Large Artery Atherosclerosis	In Situ Thrombosis	MCA Disease
33	Large Artery Atherosclerosis	In Situ Thrombosis	PCA Disease

ID	Classification	Mechanism	Specific category
34	Large Artery Atherosclerosis	In Situ Thrombosis	PCA Disease
35	Large Artery Atherosclerosis	In Situ Thrombosis	PCA Disease
36	Large Artery Atherosclerosis	In Situ Thrombosis	VA Disease
37	Large Artery Atherosclerosis	In Situ Thrombosis	PICA Disease
38	Large Artery Atherosclerosis	In Situ Thrombosis	PICA Disease
39	Large Artery Atherosclerosis	In Situ Thrombosis	PICA Disease
40	Large Artery Atherosclerosis	In Situ Thrombosis	BA Disease
41	Large Artery Atherosclerosis	In Situ Thrombosis	BA Disease
42	Large Artery Atherosclerosis	Hemodynamic	pICA Disease
43	Large Artery Atherosclerosis	Hemodynamic	pICA Disease
44	Large Artery Atherosclerosis	Hemodynamic	pICA Disease
45	Large Artery Atherosclerosis	Hemodynamic	pICA Disease
46	Large Artery Atherosclerosis	Hemodynamic	pICA Disease
47	Large Artery Atherosclerosis	Hemodynamic	dICA Disease
48	Large Artery Atherosclerosis	Hemodynamic	VA, BA Disease
49	Large Artery Atherosclerosis	Hemodynamic	Bilateral ICA Disease
50	Large Artery Atherosclerosis	Artery to Artery Embolism, In Situ Thrombosis	Combined Type
51	Large Artery Atherosclerosis	Artery to Artery Embolism, In Situ Thrombosis	Combined Type
52	Large Artery Atherosclerosis	Artery to Artery Embolism, In Situ Thrombosis	Combined Type
53	Large Artery Atherosclerosis	Artery to Artery Embolism, In Situ Thrombosis	Combined Type
54	Large Artery Atherosclerosis	Artery to Artery Embolism, In Situ Thrombosis	Combined Type
55	Large Artery Atherosclerosis	Artery to Artery Embolism, In Situ Thrombosis	Combined Type
56	Large Artery Atherosclerosis	Artery to Artery Embolism, In Situ Thrombosis	Combined Type
57	Large Artery Atherosclerosis	Artery to Artery Embolism, In Situ Thrombosis	Combined Type
58	Large Artery Atherosclerosis	Artery to Artery Embolism, Hemodynamic	Combined Type
59	Large Artery Atherosclerosis	Artery to Artery Embolism, Hemodynamic	Combined Type
60	Large Artery Atherosclerosis	Artery to Artery Embolism, Hemodynamic	Combined Type
61	Large Artery Atherosclerosis	Artery to Artery Embolism, Hemodynamic	Combined Type
62	Cadioembolism		Prosthetic Mechanical Valve
63	Cadioembolism		Prosthetic Mechanical Valve
64	Cadioembolism		Atrial Fibrillation
65	Cadioembolism		Atrial Fibrillation
66	Cadioembolism		Atrial Fibrillation

ID	Classification	Mechanism	Specific category
67		Cadioembolism	Atrial Fibrillation
68		Cadioembolism	Atrial Fibrillation
69		Cadioembolism	Atrial Fibrillation
70		Cadioembolism	Atrial Fibrillation
71		Cadioembolism	Atrial Fibrillation
72		Cadioembolism	Atrial Fibrillation
73		Cadioembolism	Atrial Fibrillation
74		Cadioembolism	Atrial Fibrillation
75		Cadioembolism	Atrial Fibrillation, Mitral Stenosis
76		Cadioembolism	Atrial Fibrillation, Mitral Stenosis
77		Cadioembolism	Atrial Fibrillation, Mitral Stenosis
78		Cadioembolism	Atrial Fibrillation/MI
79		Cadioembolism	Paroxysmal Atrial Fibrillation
80		Cadioembolism	Paroxysmal Atrial Fibrillation
81		Cadioembolism	Global Hypokinesia
82		Cadioembolism	Global Hypokinesia
83		Cadioembolism	Global Hypokinesia
84		Cadioembolism	Spontaneous Echogenic Contrast
85		Cadioembolism	Spontaneous Echogenic Contrast
86		Cadioembolism	LA Thrombi
87		Cadioembolism	PFO
88		Cadioembolism	PFO
89		Cadioembolism	PFO
90		Cadioembolism	PFO
91		Cadioembolism	PFO
92		Small Vessel Occlusion	IC Infarction
93		Small Vessel Occlusion	CR Infarction
94		Small Vessel Occlusion	CR Infarction
95		Small Vessel Occlusion	CR Infarction
96		Small Vessel Occlusion	CR Infarction
97		Small Vessel Occlusion	CR Infarction
98		Small Vessel Occlusion	CR Infarction
99		Small Vessel Occlusion	Thalamic Infarction
100		Small Vessel Occlusion	Thalamic Infarction
101		Small Vessel Occlusion	Thalamic Infarction

ID	Classification	Mechanism	Specific category
102		Small Vessel Occlusion	Pontine Infarction
103		Small Vessel Occlusion	Pontine Infarction
104		Small Vessel Occlusion	Pontine Infarction
105		Small Vessel Occlusion	Medial Medullary Infarction
106	Others	Hemodynamic	Moyamoya Disease
107	Others	Hemodynamic	Moyamoya Disease
108	Others	Hemodynamic	Moyamoya Disease
109	Others	Cadioembolism	Infective Endocarditis
110	Others	Cadioembolism	Infective Endocarditis
111	Others	Hypercoagulability	Antiphospholipid Antibody Syndrome
112	Others	Artery to Artery Embolism	Post-Radiotherapy Complication
113	Others	Artery to Artery Embolism	Arterial Dissection
114	Others	In Situ Thrombosis	Arterial Dissection
115	Others	In Situ Thrombosis	Arterial Dissection
116	Others	Artery to Artery Embolism	Arterial Dissection
117	Others	Paradoxical Embolism	Pulmonary Arteriovenous Fistula
118	Others	Hypercoagulability	Cancer
119	Others	Cadioembolism	Coronary Artery Bypass Graft Surgery
120	Others	Venous Thrombosis	Cerebral Venous Thrombosis
121	Others	Venous Thrombosis	Cerebral Venous Thrombosis
122	Others	Hypercoagulability	Thrombotic Thrombocytopenic Purpura
123	Others	Artery to Artery Embolism, Hemodynamic	Takayasu's Arteritis
124	Others	Unknown	CADASIL
125	Others	Unknown	CADASIL
126	Others	Unknown	MELAS
127	Others	Unknown	MELAS
128	Others	Unknown	MELAS
129	Others	Congenital	ICA Agenesis
130	Others	Unknown	Hyperhomocysteinemia
131	Others	Unknown	Hypertensive Encephalopathy
132		Cadioembolism	Postischemic Hyperperfusion
133	Large Artery Atherosclerosis	Artery to Artery Embolism	Malignant Infarction
134	Large Artery Atherosclerosis	In Situ Thrombosis	Dominant ACA
135	Undetermined	Negative	DWI-PWI Mismatch

ID	Classification	Mechanism	Specific category
136	Large Artery Atherosclerosis	Artery to Artery Embolism	Contralateral Infarction
137	Large Artery Atherosclerosis	Artery to Artery Embolism	Medial Medulla+Cerebellar Infarction
138	Cadioembolism		Hemorrhage Signal on GRE
139	Large Artery Atherosclerosis	Artery to Artery Embolism	Lateral Thalamic Infarction
140	Large Artery Atherosclerosis	In Situ Thrombosis	Basilar Stenosis
141	Brain Edema	Venous Thrombosis	Cerebral Venous Thrombosis
142	Small Vessel Occlusion		Concomitant ICH
143	Large Artery Atherosclerosis	Artery to Artery Embolism	Retinal Artery Occlusion
144	Large Artery Atherosclerosis	Artery to Artery Embolism	Basilar Artery Dolichoectasia
145	Large Artery Atherosclerosis	Artery to Artery Embolism, In Situ Thrombosis	Locked-In Syndrome
146	Large Artery Atherosclerosis	Vertebrobasilar Insufficiency	Subclavian Steal Syndrome
147	Large Artery Atherosclerosis	Hemodynamic	Angioplasty-Induced Hypoperfusion
148	Undetermined	Negative	Concomitant ICH
149	Large Artery Atherosclerosis	Artery to Artery Embolism	Concomitant ICH
150	Cadioembolism		Malignant MCA Infarction
151	Large Artery Atherosclerosis		Imaging Follow-Up after Intracranial Stent
152	Large Artery Atherosclerosis	Artery to Artery Embolism, In Situ Thrombosis	Malignant Cerebellar Infarction
153	Cadioembolism		Anticoagulation Time
154	Large Artery Atherosclerosis	Artery to Artery Embolism	Microembolic Signals on TCD
155	Large Artery Atherosclerosis	Artery to Artery Embolism	Ulcerative Plaque
156	Cadioembolism		Malignant Cerebellar Infarction
157	Large Artery Atherosclerosis	Artery to Artery Embolism	Tandem Lesion
158	Large Artery Atherosclerosis	Artery to Artery Embolism	Intracranial Angioplasty
159	Large Artery Atherosclerosis	Hemodynamic	ECA Angioplasty
160	Large Artery Atherosclerosis	Hemodynamic	Angioplasty-Induced Hypoperfusion
161	Large Artery Atherosclerosis	Hemodynamic	Hyperperfusion Syndrome
162	Large Artery Atherosclerosis	Artery to Artery Embolism	Post-Stent Embolism
163	Large Artery Atherosclerosis	Artery to Artery Embolism	Synkinesis
164	Small Vessel Occlusion		Uncrossed Corticospinal Tract Lesion
165	Cadioembolism		Functional Takeover Phenomenon
166	Small Vessel Occlusion		Cortical Reorganization
167	Small Vessel Occlusion		Cortical Reorganization

LIST OF ABBREVIATIONS

ACA: Anterior Cerebral Artery

Acom: Anterior Communicating Artery

ADC: Apparent Diffusion Coefficient

AICA: Anterior Inferior Cerebellar Artery

ASA: Anterior Spinal Artery

ASO: Atherosclerosis Obliterans

AVM: Arteriovenous Malformation

BA: Basilar Artery

BP: Blood Pressure

CABG: Coronary Artery Bypass Surgery

CADASIL: Cerebral Autosomal Dominant Arteriopathy with Subcortical Infarcts and Leukoencephalopathy

CBV: Cerebral Blood Volume

CCA: Common Carotid Artery

CEA: Carotid Endarterectomy

CSF: Cerebral Spinal Fluid

CT: Computed Tomography

DWI: Diffusion-Weighted Image

ECA: External Carotid Artery

ECG: Electrocardiography

EEG: Electroencephalography

EDAS: Encephaloduroarteriosynangiosis

FDP: Fibrin Degradation Product

FLAIR: Fluid-Attenuated Inversion Recovery

GRE: Gradient Echo

ICA: Internal Cerebral Artery

ICU: Intensive Care Unit

IICP: Increased Intracranial Pressure

INR: International Normalized Ratio

LVH: Left Ventricular Hypertrophy

MCA: Middle Cerebral Artery

MELAS: Mitochondrial Myopathy, Encephalopathy, Lactic Acidosis, and Stroke

MRA: Magnetic Resonance Angiography
MRI: Magnetic Resonance Image
MRC: Medical Research Counsil
NIHSS: National Institute of Health Stroke Scale
OA: Ophthalmic Artery
PCA: Posterior Cerebral Artery
Pcom: Posterior Communicating Artery
PFO: Patent Foramen Ovale
PICA: Posterior Inferior Cerebellar Artery
PLED: Periodic Lateralized Epileptiform Discharge
PT: Prothrombin Time
PVWM: Periventricular White Matter
SCA: Superior Cerebellar Artery
SPECT: Single Photon Emission Computed Tomography
STA: Superficial Temporal Artery
rt-PA: Recombinant Tissue Plasminogen Activator
T2WI: T2-Weighted Image
TCD: Transcranial Doppler
TOAST: Trial of ORG 10172 in Acute Stroke Treatment
TOF: Time of Flight
TFCA: Transfemoral Cerebral Angiography
VA: Vertebral Artery
VPL: Ventral Postero Lateral Nucleus

I

Stroke Mechanisms

1. Large Artery Atherosclerosis
2. Cardioembolism
3. Small Vessel Occlusion
4. Other Atypical Causes

Ischemic stroke develops when there is an interruption of cerebral blood flow to an area of the brain, and this may result from large artery atherosclerosis, cardioembolism, small vessel or penetrating artery diseases, non-atherosclerotic arteriopathies, hypercoagulable states of various disorders, and genetic or metabolic disorders. General stroke mechanisms are usually determined by the Trial of ORG 10172 in Acute Stroke Treatment (TOAST) criteria: large artery atherosclerosis, cardioembolism, and small vessel occlusion.[1] For further understanding of ischemic stroke mechanisms, I subdivided the large artery atherosclerosis into artery to artery embolism, low flow stroke, and thrombosis in situ. The manual for stroke subtyping is described in the Korean Stroke Registry website (http://www.strokedb.or.kr). This classification of stroke subtypes helps us understand the stroke mechanisms more clearly and allows us to treat patients with confidence, but it is sometimes difficult to establish the cause because of the frequent overlapping of the subtypes and non-specific radiological findings.

1. Large Artery Atherosclerosis

The diagnosis of large artery atherosclerosis requires the evidence of an atherosclerotic lesion involving the intracranial or extracranial large arteries (stenosis ≥ 50% or vulnerable plaques) which supply blood to the area of infarction. The distribution of cerebral atherosclerosis is different in certain ethnic groups, although it also depends on life style. Stenosis of major intracranial arteries is more prevalent among Asians than in whites, while extracranial artery stenosis is more prevalent in whites. Stroke associated with large artery atherosclerosis usually occur in patients with significant risk factors for atherosclerosis. Patients with large artery atherosclerosis stroke are also at high risk for the development of other vascular complications. The mechanisms of large artery atherosclerosis stroke reflect various plaque complications including intraplaque hemorrhage, extensive necrosis, inflammation, calcification, or thrombosis in the underlying arterial stenosis. Large artery atherosclerosis is composed of artery-to-artery embolization, in situ thrombosis, hemodynamic, and combined type. Artery-to-artery embolism is the most common mechanism of large artery atherosclerosis stroke. Proximal and distal internal carotid artery, proximal and distal vertebral artery, major intra-cranial artery stems around the circle of Willis, basilar artery, and occasionally the aortic arch are the main embolic sources. Ruptured, ulcerated or thrombosed extracranial or major intracranial atherosclerotic plaques frequently induce an artery-to-artery embolism. The subtype of artery-to-artery embolism is easily confirmed if multiple cortical lesions or a single territory lesion is seen on diffusion-weighted images (DWI) in the brain areas supplied by the relevant proximal intracranial or extracranial atherosclerotic arteries which also can be seen by another imaging technique, magnetic resonance angiography (MRA) [Fig 1a]. In situ thrombosis reflects thrombosis or plaque disruption in the setting of pre-existing arterial stenosis, subsequently compromising blood flow to the nearby penetrating arteries. In situ thrombosis frequently occurs in the middle cerebral artery stems, distal vertebral arteries, proximal posterior cerebral arteries and basilar artery [Fig. 1b]. Hemodynamic alterations (low flow strokes) also may trigger ischemic injury in the watershed area of a tight stenotic artery. The hemodynamic mechanism is based on a history of low-flow events such as dehydration, hypotension, hot bathing, drinking, postprandial conditions, or symptoms that occur during orthostatic conditions such as limb-shaking paralysis, etc., and radiological evidence of borderzone lesions between the main branching arterial supplies of a proximal culprit arterial lesion, usually proximal ICA or rarely MCA stem [Fig 1c]. Combined types include two or more of the afore-mentioned mechanisms, which may have a perforator zone infarction due to an in situ thrombosis and an artery to artery distal pial artery zone infarction or a border zone infarction caused by low flow [Fig. 1d].

The author would like to mention transient ischemic attacks (TIA) here. TIA is one of the clinical types of ischemic stroke in which symptoms last less than 24 hours. TIA can be further classified as embolic and low flow type TIAs in patients with large artery atherosclerosis, and TIAs of small vessel disease. Embolic TIA is much more common than low flow type TIA, and its symptoms manifest by embolization of a thrombus from the proximal atheromatous artery to a distal branch and disappear following the lysis of the embolus. Embolic TIAs of a long duration usually tend to have lesions visualized by DWI, whereas TIAs of a short duration that resolve within several minutes typically do not have DWI lesions. The usual duration of TIAs is short, lasting a few minutes to half an hour. On the other hand, low flow TIAs tend to have longer duration and no DWI lesions because the low flow effect on the brain tissue is sub-lethal in intensity and duration. When the low-flow ischemic degree is severe and the duration is long, then there could be diffusion abnormality.

Figure 1. Schema of Large Artery Atherosclerosis Subtype

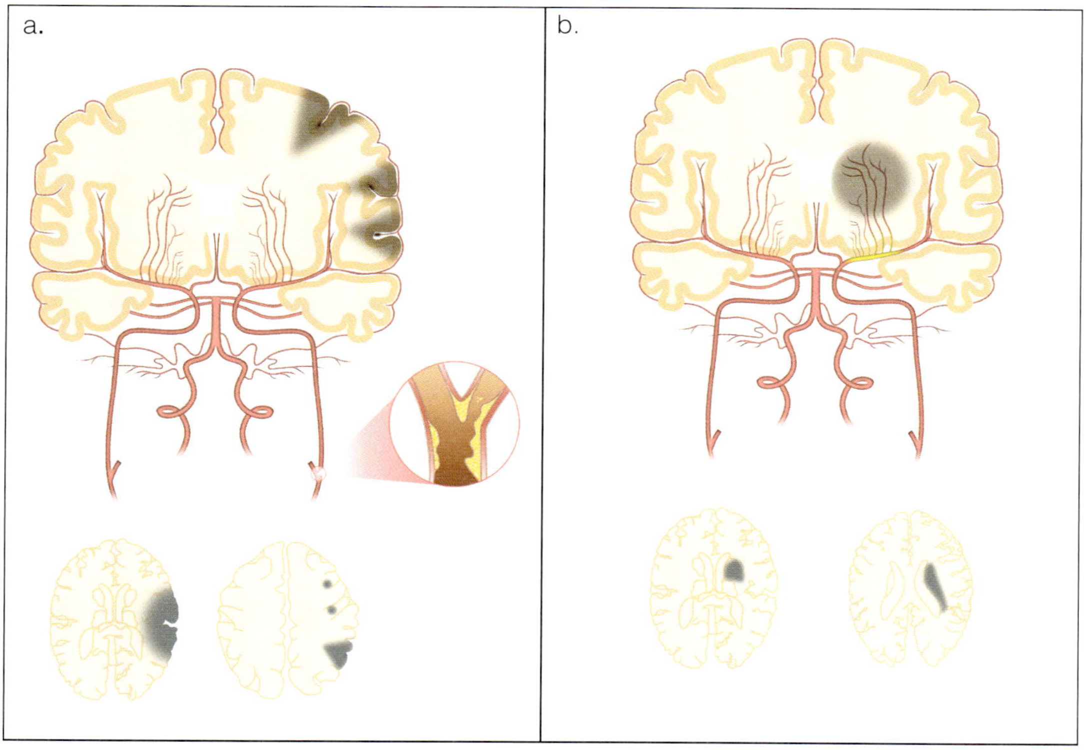

c.

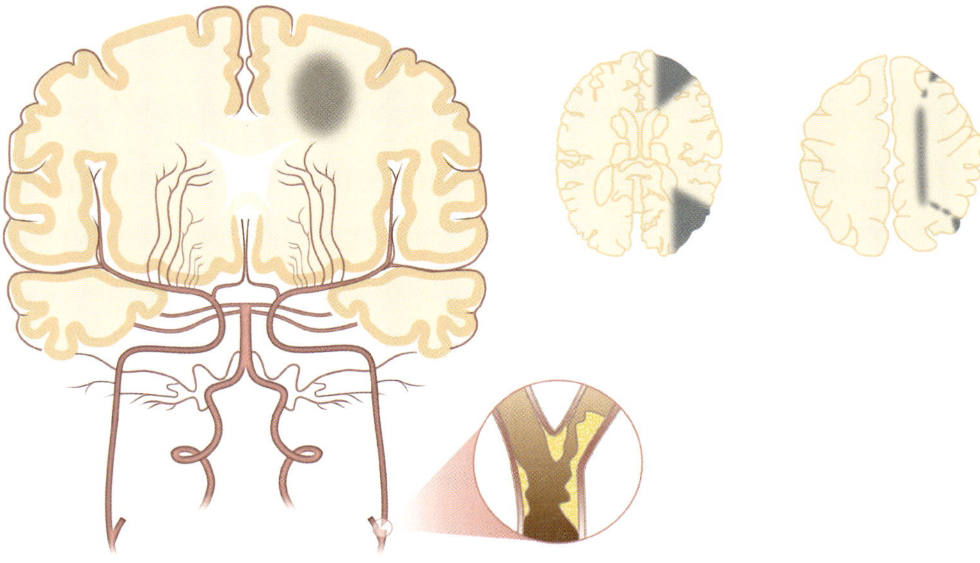

d.

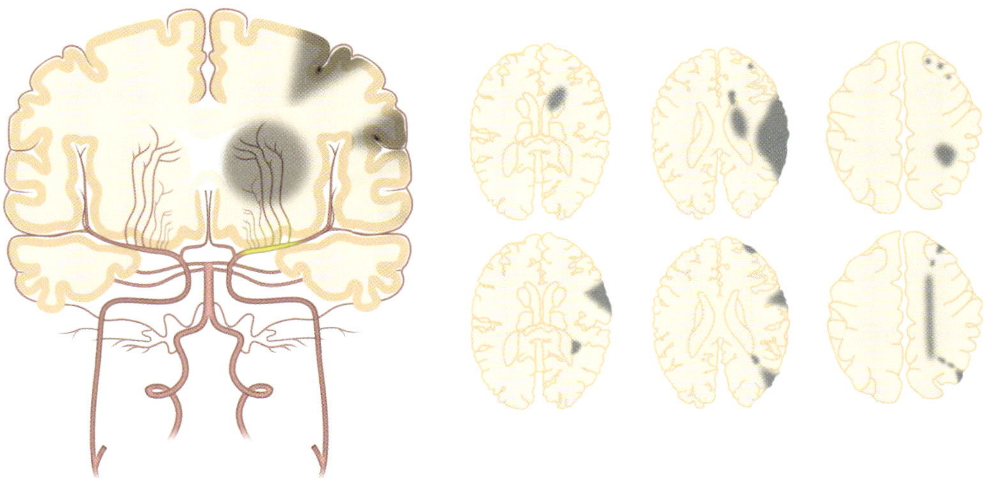

2. Cardioembolism

Ischemic stroke is a serious complication in patients with cardiac disorders. Cardioembolisms account for about 20% of all ischemic strokes.[2] The most common cause of cardioembolic strokes in older patients is nonvalvular atrial fibrillation, which accounts for two-thirds of cases. Other high risk groups include patients with acute myocardial infarction, mitral or aortic valve disease, mechanical prosthetic valves, sick sinus syndrome, dilated or congestive cardiomyopathies, infective endocarditis, and atrial myxomas (Table 1).[2] Cardioembolic infarcts are often large wedge-shaped, multiple, bilateral, or hemorrhagic [Fig. 2]. Cardioembolism is suspected if the patient is at high-risk to develop stroke from cardiogenic source. However, clinical determination of cardioembolic stroke is sometimes difficult, even if a potential cardioembolic source is identified. Many cardiac problems may coexist with cerebral atherosclerosis, and atrial fibrillation may occur just after an ischemic stroke. Clinical manifestations and radiological findings should be considered as well as the identification of a potential embolic source. Radiologically, the brain parenchyma in cardioembolic stroke has fewer T2 high signal lesions than stroke caused by vascular factors, and cardiogenic embolic infarctions tend to undergo hemorrhagic transformation.

Figure 2. Schema of Cardioembolism Subtype

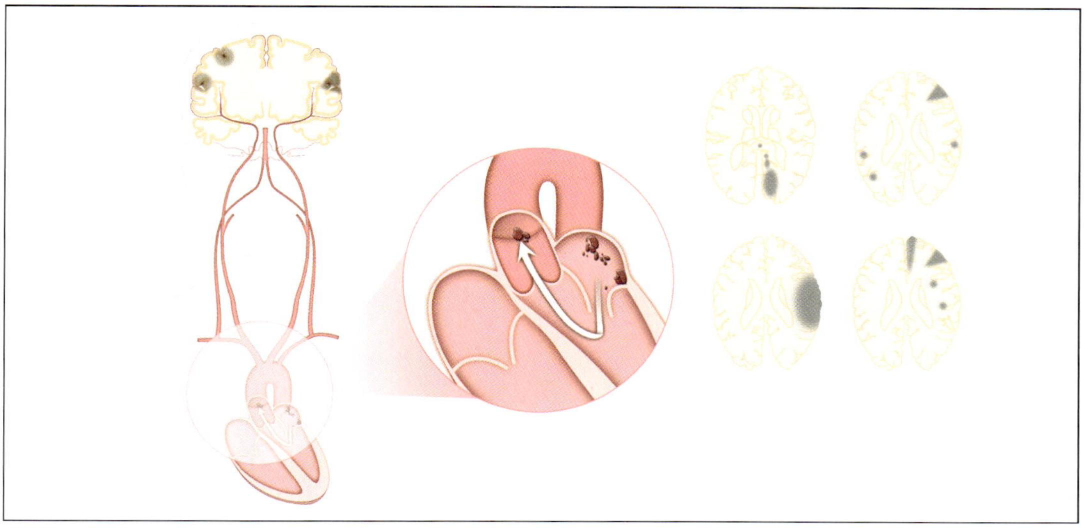

Table 1. Potential Carodioembolic Sources

Definite Risk	Possible/Probable Risk
Atrial fibrillation	Patent foramen ovale
Sustained atrial flutter	Atrial septal aneurysm
Sick sinus syndrome	Atrial or ventricular septal defects
Atrial myxoma	Spontaneous echocontrast in left atrial appendage
Left atrial appendage thrombus	Subaortic hypertrophic cardiomyopathy
Recent myocardial infarction	Mitral valve prolapsed
Left ventricular akinesia	Calcified aortic stenosis
Left ventricular thrombus	Valve strands
Dilated cardiomyopathy	Fibroelastoma
Prosthetic heart valve	
Rheumatic mitral stenosis	
Infective endocarditis	

3. Small Vessel Occlusion

Small vessel or penetrating artery disease, namely lacunes, usually develops in patients with long-standing, poorly-controlled arterial hypertension, diabetes mellitus, and current smokers. The diagnosis of strokes caused by small vessel occlusions is based on the size (less than 1.5cm in diameter) and location of the ischemic lesions within the penetrator zones. But the author, personally, thinks that the size should be extend to less than 2cm on DWI because the final lesion can shrink to less than 1.5cm. Pathologically structural changes of the cerebral arterioles caused by hypertension are characterized by lipohyalinosis, microaneurysm formation, and fibrinoid necrosis. The endothelial damage of the small penetrating arteries, microatheroma of the penetrating artery, embolism, and hemorrheological disturbances are possibly etiologies in lacunar infarctions. The infarctions occur in the regions supplied by the small penetrating arteries. The basal ganglia, pons, thalamus, internal capsule, and corona radiata are the most frequent sites [Fig. 3a, b]. Sometimes, a lacune occurs by the atherosclerotic change of the parent artery invoving the orifice of a penetrator [Fig. 3c]. In this case, the stroke mechanism is thought to be an in situ thrombosis, but its clinical entity is still a lacune or a small vessel disease in

TOAST classification. Multiple lacunar infarctions are frequently associated with cerebral microbleeds, leukoaraiosis, and intracerebral hemorrhage, which are also end organ damage markers of chronic hypertension. In general, for the diagnosis of small vessel occlusion strokes, other causes of ischemic stroke should be ruled out, because they are frequently accompanied by other atherosclerotic and cardiac disorders. Lacunar stroke has several clinical entities: pure motor hemiparesis which is the most common type and has lesions in the motor pathways (the corona radiata, internal capsule, pontine base, and rarely the medullary pyramis); pure sensory stroke which has lesions in the thalamus, mainly in ventral posterolateral nucleus (VPL) and rarely in the thalamo-cortical projections; ataxic hemiparesis which has lesions involving both pyramidal and frontopontocerebellar tracts in the internal capsule, corona radiata, and upper pons; sensorimotor stroke which is rare and has lesions involving both sensory and motor pathways by a indistinct penetrator vascular territory; and dysarthria clumsy hand syndrome which has lesions near the genu of the internal capsule or upper pons, and other rare conditions.

Figure 3. Schema of Small Vessel Occlusion Subtype

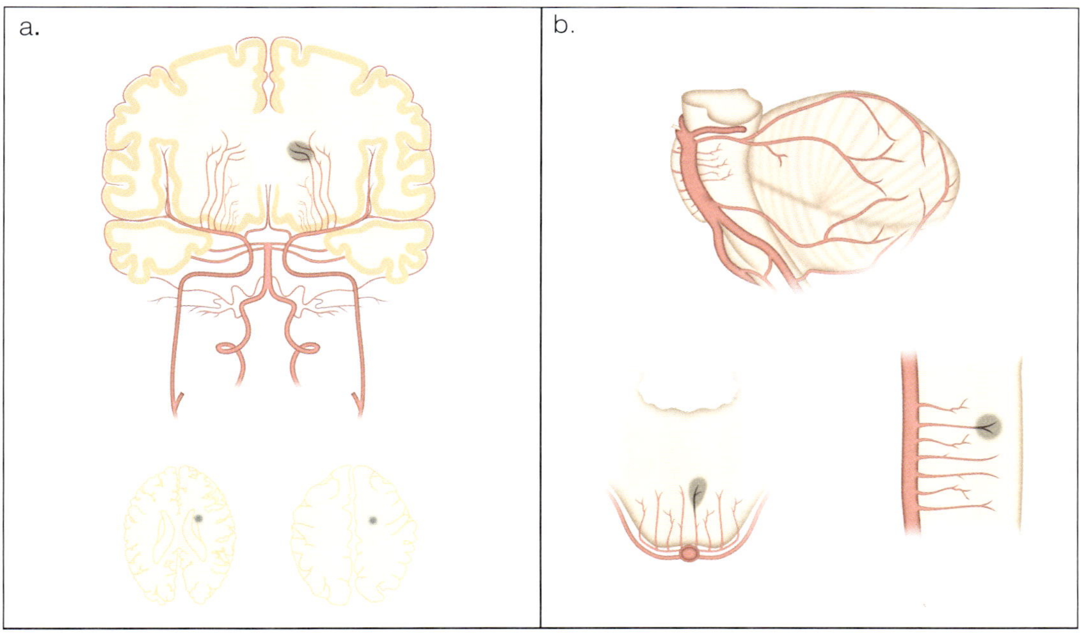

C.

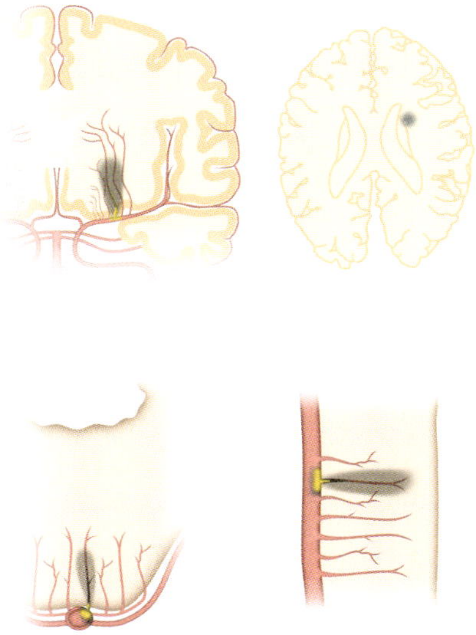

4. Other Atypical Causes

Although the majority of ischemic strokes are induced by the above three causes, several non-atherosclerotic vasculopathies can be responsible for a minority of ischemic strokes. These specific categories include arterial dissection, Moyamoya disease, cerebral vasculitis, radiation vasculopathies, hypercoagulable disorders, and genetic or metabolic disorders (Table 2).[3,4] These specific conditions should be considered in young patients with ischemic or hemorrhagic stroke, patients with a definite family history, patients with recurrent strokes, and patients with strokes associated with chronic progressive neurological symptoms. When there is no definite history of common vascular risk factors in stroke and/or there is no typical vascular territorial involvement in radiologic findings, these atypical causes should also be differentiated.

Table 2. Atypical Disorders Causing Cerebral Infarction

Nonatherosclerotic Vasculopathies	Inherited and Miscellaneous Disorders	Hypercoagulable Disorders
Arterial dissection	Moyamoya disease	Antithrombin III deficiency
Radiation-induced vasculopathy	MELAS	Protein C, S deficiency
Migrainous infarction	CADASIL	Factor V leiden mutation
Cerebral vasculitis	Fibromuscular dysplasia	Antiphopholipid antibody syndrome
Infectious vasculitis	Homocystinuria	Malignancy
Necrotizing vasculitis	Fabry's disease	Pregnancy
Polyarteritis nodosa	Marfan's syndrome	Oral contraceptives
Wegener's granulomatosis	Ehlers-Danlos syndrome	Polycythemia vera
Churg-Strauss syndrome		Essential thrombocythemia
Collagen vascular disease		Thrombotic thrombocytopenic purpura
Systemic lupus erythematosus		Chemotherapeutic agents
Rheumatoid arthritis		
Scleroderma		
Sjogren's syndrome		
Giant cell arteritis		
Takayasu's arteritis		
Temporal arteritis		
Hypersensitiivty vasculitis		
Henoch-Schonlein purpura		
Drug-induced vasculitis		
Sarcoidosis		
Behcet's disease		
Ulcerative colitis		

II

Typical Mechanisms

1. Large Artery Atherosclerosis

2. Cardioembolism

3. Small Vessel Occlusion

1. Large Artery Atherosclerosis

1-1. Artery to Artery Embolism

• Case 1

A 56-year-old man presented with a sudden paresthesia in his left lower limb. He was a heavy smoker of 40 packyears. He had no history of hypertension, diabetes mellitus, and hypercholesterolemia. He had no family history or previous history of stroke. Visual field examination showed a left inferior quadrantanopsia. There was no motor or visual neglect on the left side. His left lower extremity was mildly weak (MRC grade IV+), while his upper extremity was intact. He also had ipsilateral sensory loss of his leg. Investigations for systemic vasculitis, coagulation abnormalities and cardioembolic sources revealed no remarkable findings. Transesophageal echocardiography showed an atherosclerotic plaque of the aortic arch.

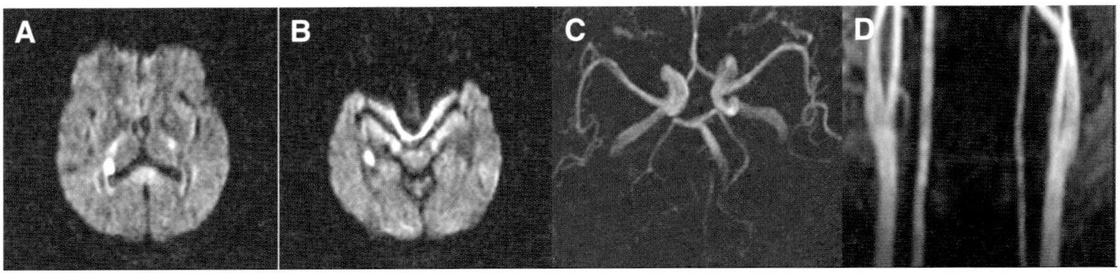

Brain MR-DWI (A, B) showed small infarcts in the right lateral thalamus, far posterior limb of internal capsule and deep medial temporal lobe. Brain MRA showed no definite stenosis or occlusions in the intracranial (C) and extracranial arteries (D). He was treated with an antiplatelet agent. His neurological symptoms improved steadily.

The involvement of the territory of the anterior choroidal artery is frequently associated with a cardioembolism of the territory of the internal carotid artery.[5] This patient has an atheroma on the aortic arch, which was verified by transesophageal echocardiography. The stroke mechanism was an artery to artery embolism from aortic arch to the right anterior choroidal artery.

• Case 2

A 67-year-old woman visited us because of a sudden visual disturbance and headache of 3 days. There were no motor or sensory symptoms. She had no history of hypertension, dyslipidemia, trauma, seizure or diabetes mellitus. She was alert and oriented with intact cognitive function. Visual field examination showed left homonymous hemianopsia. There was no motor or visual neglect on the left side. Prosopagnosia was absent. Cranial nerve examinations were normal. Motor and sensory examinations showed no abnormal findings. Ataxia, tremor and gait abnormality were not noted. Investigations for coagulation abnormalities, systemic vasculitis and cardioembolic sources showed no remarkable findings. Transesophageal echocardiography revealed moderate atherosclerosis at aortic arch.

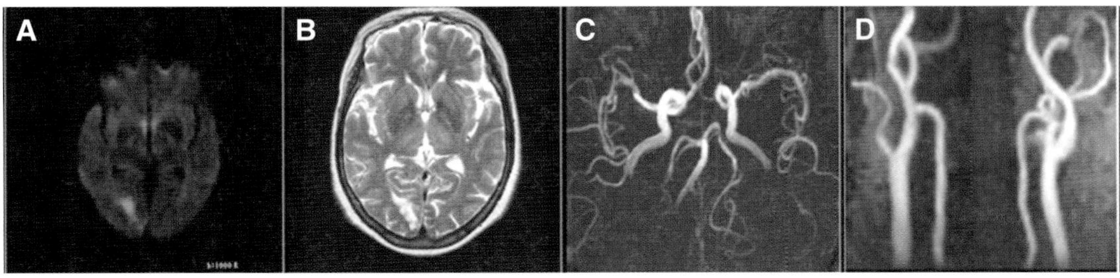

Brain MR-DWI (A, B) showed a right PCA infarct. Brain MRA (C, D) showed mild right P2 stenosis, hypoplastic left A1 and intact extracranial cerebral arteries. The patient was treated with dual antiplatelet agents.

An unstable atherosclerotic plaque on the aortic arch can release embolisms into anterior and posterior circulation. In this case, the stroke mechanism seemed to be an embolic infarct from aortic arch to the right PCA.

• Case 3

A 76-year-old man was hospitalized because of a sudden left-sided weakness, which had developed 2 days before admission. He had no dysarthria, dysphagia, and other neurologic deficits. 10 years before, he had been diagnosed with a left PICA infarction and was taking aspirin. He had hypertension. The motor power of the left limbs was all MRC grade IV. The cerebellar function test showed mild dysmetria of the left limbs. Echocardiography showed mild concentric LVH and aortic valve sclerosis but were otherwise within normal limits.

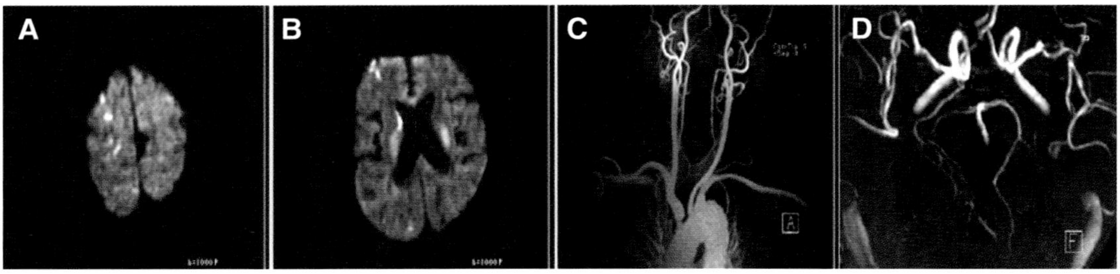

Brain MR-DWI (A, B) showed multiple infarctions involving the right ACA, MCA and PCA territories. Extracranial brain MRA (C) showed significant focal stenosis of the orifice of the right CCA (arrow), and intracranial MRA (D) showed multiple irregular stenoses of the right A1 artery, both MCA bifurcations, and fetal circulation of the right PCA. We started dual antiplatelet agents, and his symptoms improved.

The stroke mechanism might be an artery to artery embolism from the right proximal CCA to the right ACA, MCA and PCA territories via fetal circulation. Hemorrheologic factors or anatomic variations could contribute to the pathogenesis of the acute multiple infarctions in both cerebral hemispheres or in both anterior and posterior circulations. The causes of acute multiple infarctions on MRI according to the vascular tree in particular cases have already been well described by the author et al.[6]

• Case 4

An 80-year-old man was admitted to the neurology ward because of a sudden right lower leg weakness that developed 1 day ago. Dysarthria and sensory changes were absent. He had a previous stroke presenting with right arm weakness 8 months ago. Other stroke risk factors included hyperlipidemia, hypertension and smoking. Mental state and cranial nerve examinations were normal. His right leg weakness was an MRC grade IV. Right knee jerk was hyperreflexive and right Babinski sign was positive. On transesophageal echocardiography, there was a protruding atheroma in the descending aorta and aortic arch.

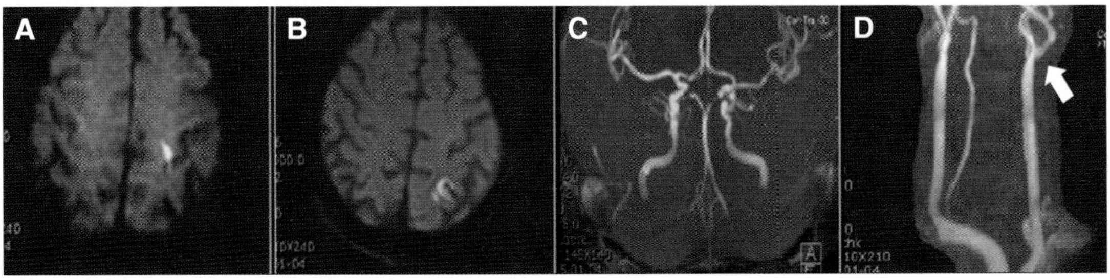

There was a small acute infarction in left fronto-parietal convexity 8 months ago (A). A new, small, acute infarction was detected in the left fronto-parietal high convexity in the current brain MR-DWI (B). There was no significant stenosis on the intracranial arteries on brain MRA (C). Contrast-MRA showed mild stenosis of the left proximal ICA (D). We had treated the patient with aspirin since the first stroke. After the second stroke, we added clopidogrel. His right leg weakness improved gradually.

The mechanism of ischemic stroke in this patient was thought to be an artery to artery embolism from the left proximal ICA or aortic arch to pial branches of the left MCA.

• Case 5

A 76-year-old man was admitted because of a left-sided weakness. He had suffered from hypertension since 10 years before the current admission, and had taken regular medication. He had no history of diabetes mellitus, heart disease, or previous stroke. He was alert and oriented with intact cognitive function. There was no motor or visual neglect on the left side. Cranial nerve examinations were normal except for mild dysarthria. His left upper extremity was weak (MRC grade IV-). Sensory examination showed no abnormal findings. Ataxia, tremor and gait abnormality were not noted. Transthoracic echocardiography and Holter monitoring did not reveal any cardiac source of embolism.

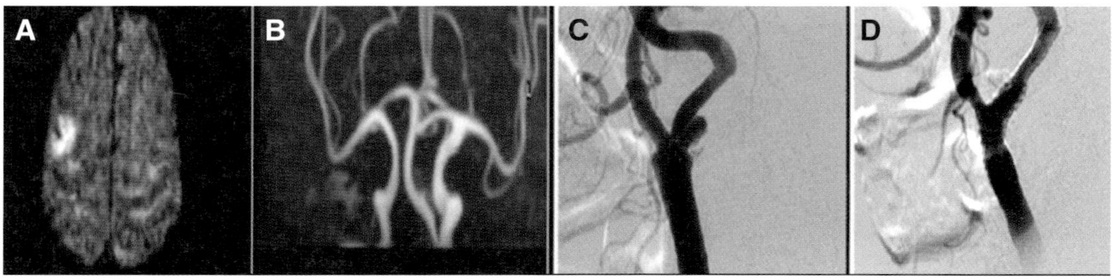

Brain MR-DWI (A) showed multiple lesions in the right frontal cortex. Brain MRA (B) showed no significant steno-occlusive lesions of the intracranial arteries. Conventional angiography (C) showed moderate stenosis with ulceration of the right proximal ICA. He was treated with dual antiplatelet agents. His neurological symptoms fully improved. 1 month later, a stent was inserted in the right proximal ICA (D).

The stroke mechanism was an artery to artery embolism from the right proximal ICA to a pial branch of the right MCA.

• Case 6

A 72-year-old man visited our hospital complaining of a sudden language disturbance and right-sided weakness. He had a history of gastrectomy for gastric cancer and hypertension for which he was taking regular medication. However, he denied having diabetes mellitus, heart disease and hypercholesterolemia. He was an ex-smoker with a history of 20 packyears. Upon visiting hospital, his BP was 150/80mmHg. His mental state was alert, but a language function test showed global aphasia. On cranial nerve examination, a central-type right facial palsy and dysphagia were noticed. Motor power of the upper extremity was MRC grade II and the lower extremity was MRC grade IV on the right side. Sensation to pain was decreased on the right side. Deep tendon reflexes were increased on the right side. Serum laboratory results, ECG, and transthoracic echocardiography were normal.

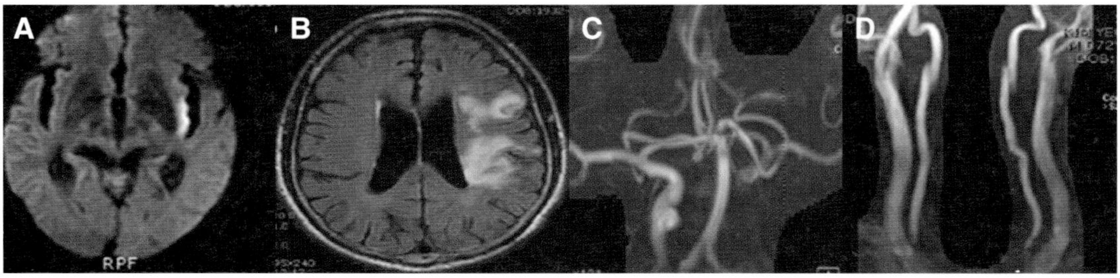

Brain MRI (A, B) showed large multifocal ischemic infarctions in the left frontal, temporal, and parietal lobes and the left insular area. Complete occlusion of the left ICA at the proximal portion was seen on brain MRA (C, D), but collateral circulation of the left ACA and MCA from the contralateral right carotid and vertebral systems were good. He was treated with an antiplatelet agent, and his symptoms slowly improved.

The mechanism of stroke was thought to be artery to artery embolism somewhere (distal stump or tight stenotic atheroma) from the non-visible left ICA. Brain MRA revealed an occlusion of the left ICA but blood flow through the left ICA was detected on TCD. The term "atheromatous pseudoocclusion" of the ICA has been described as an extreme type of stenosing lesion which is misdiagnosed as a complete occlusion during non-invasive procedures.[7] Its recognition requires special sonographic and angiographic techniques.

• Case 7

A 73-year-old man was admitted with right-sided weakness that developed 1 day ago. He presented with dysarthria, language disturbance and drowsy mentality. Medical history revealed hypertension and diabetes mellitus. His mental status was drowsy. Cranial nerve examination revealed a right central facial palsy and dysarthria. The motor power on the right side was MRC grade III-IV. His cerebellar function was uncheckable. Carotid and ophthalmic bruits were inaudible. His FBS and HbA1c were 210mg/dL and 8.1%, respectively. The echocardiographic examination showed a protruding atheroma in ascending aortic arch. There was no embolic source in the intracardiac areas. Holter monitoring showed only atrial tachycardia.

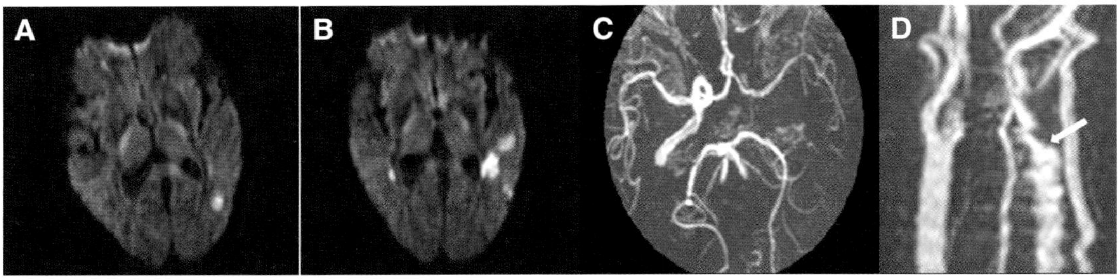

Brain MR-DWI (A, B) showed multiple infarctions in both cerebral hemispheres. Left proximal ICA occlusion (arrow) was observed on brain MRA (C, D). Severe stenosis of the right proximal ICA was also noted (D). Aspirin was started initially; however, 10 days after onset, his right-sided weakness aggravated along with fever and pneumonia. A follow-up MRI showed newly developed multiple infarctions. Thereafter, the treatment regimen was changed to an anticoagulant.

The stroke mechanism might be an artery to artery embolism from the right proximal ICA or aortic arch to the right MCA (a small deep temporal lesion) and to the left MCA (multiple temporal lesions) possibly through the Acom.

• Case 8

A 67-year-old man had a sudden weakness of the left side, which was accompanied by mental deterioration. The weakness was near hemiplegia. His past medical history included hypertension that was diagnosed 2 years ago and smoking of 40 packyears. His mental status was drowsy. He had a gaze preponderance to the right and left homonymous hemianopsia. He had dysarthria and dysphagia. His motor power on the left side was an MRC grade I with a positive Babinski sign, and hypesthesia of the left side was also observed. Echocardiography and Holter monitoring showed no abnormal findings.

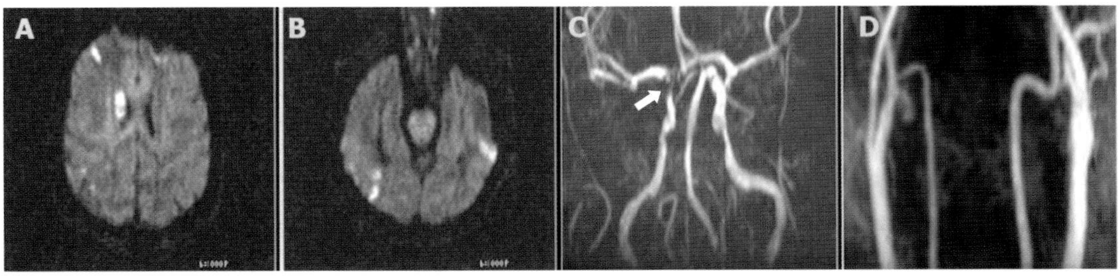

He visited our hospital 1.5 hours after the onset of symptoms, and intravenous thrombolysis with rt-PA was done. MR-DWI (A, B) showed multiple infarctions involving the right MCA territory. MRA (C, D) showed severe stenosis of the right supraclinoid ICA (arrow), and mild diffuse luminal narrowings. His initial NIHSS was 23, and after a few hours, the NIHSS was 6. And at discharge, the NIHSS was 0.

He had a history of hypertension and smoking. Images revealed a right MCA infarction with ICA and PCA stenosis. The stroke mechanism was thought to be an artery to artery embolism from the right distal ICA lodging into the MCA perforator zone initially and then disrupting into the pial artery territories.

• Case 9

A 43-year-old woman presented with recurrent, transient numbness in the right face and arm. The symptoms developed 5 times over 3 days with the same nature and lasted 5 to 10 minutes. She had hypercholesterolemia and was taking medication irregularly. She had no history of hypertension and diabetes mellitus. She had no family or previous history of stroke. There was no language disturbance. Cranial examinations were normal. Motor and sensory examinations showed no abnormal findings. Cholesterol level was 278mg/dL. Investigations for systemic vasculitis and coagulation abnormalities and echocardiography revealed no remarkable findings.

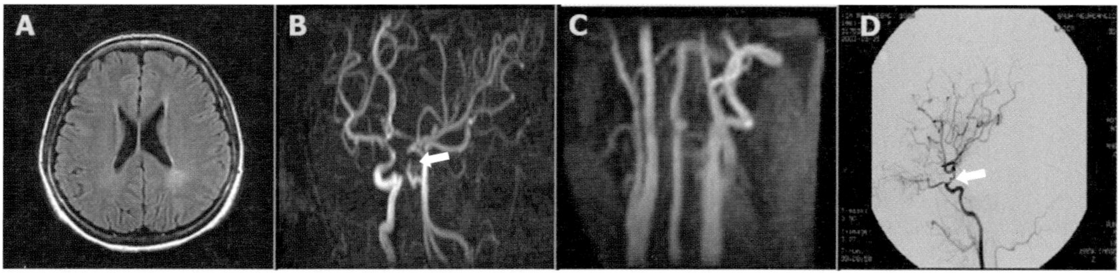

On brain MR-DWI, there was no evidence of acute infarct. However, FLAIR imaging (A) showed a high signal intensity lesion in the left peritrigonal area. Brain MRA (B, C) and TFCA (D) showed a severe stenosis of the left supraclinoid ICA (arrows). She was treated with an antiplatelet agent and statin, and thereafter she had no further symptoms.

Since there was no definite history of dehydration or hypotension at time of the attacks and no further attacks occurred after medication, the stroke mechanism was thought to be a diffusion-negative TIA due to an artery to artery embolism. The high signal intensity lesion in the deep parietal (peritrigonal) area of the FLAIR image was not thought to be directly related to the patient's symptoms, but suggested longstanding ischemic damage due to the tight distal ICA stenosis. Embolic TIAs of long duration usually have lesions on DWI, whereas shorter TIAs do not necessarily have any. On the other hand, TIAs of low flow usually have no DWI positive lesions.

• Case 10

A 66-year-old woman presented with a sudden right-sided weakness and language disturbance on the day of visit. 10 years before admission, she had a left-sided weakness and recovered fully after 1 month. At that time, hypertension had been detected, but was poorly controlled thereafter. She had no history of diabetes mellitus or heart disease. She was alert but showed motor aphasia. Cranial nerve examination showed no abnormal findings except a right facial palsy of the central type and dysarthria. Her motor power of the right side was an MRC grade IV. Sensory examination also showed right hypesthesia. Echocardiographic examination showed no remarkable abnormal findings except concentric LVH.

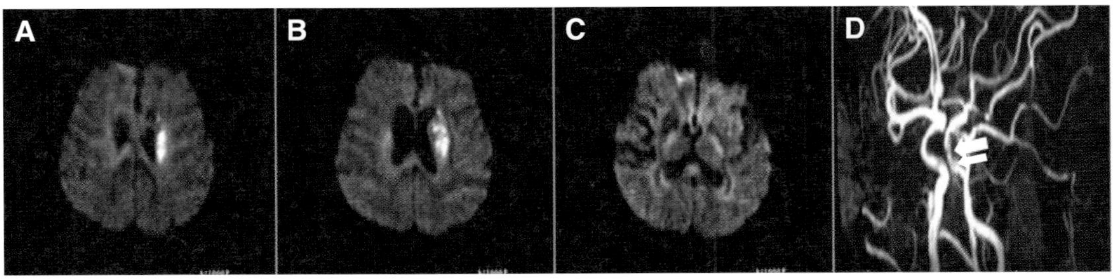

Brain MR-DWI (A-C) showed an acute infarct in the left basal ganglia. MRA (D) revealed a stenosis in the left distal ICA (arrow). She was treated with aspirin.

The stroke mechanism was thought to be an artery to artery embolism from the left distal ICA to the perforator zone of the MCA stem.

• Case 11

A 71-year-old man presented with a sudden weakness of his right upper extremity and aphasia which developed after a prostatectomy under general anesthesia. He had a partial gastrectomy 10 years ago and hypertension for 7 years. On neurologic examination, there was motor aphasia, a right upper extremity weakness (MRC grade III) and a right central-type facial palsy. Echocardiography showed inferior wall hypokinesia.

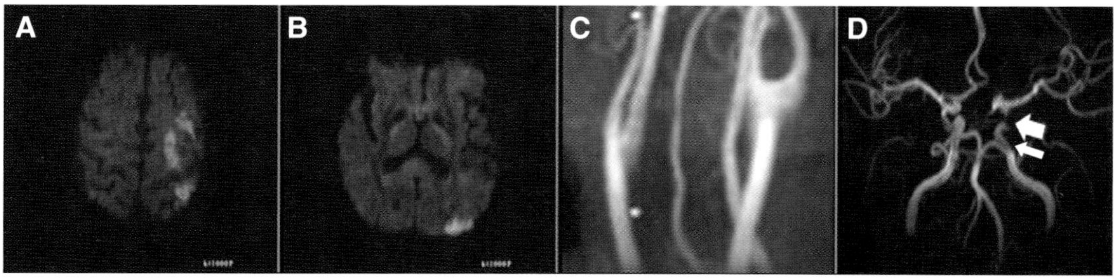

Brain MR-DWI (A, B) showed multiple left MCA territory infarctions. Brain MRA (C, D) revealed a severe left distal ICA stenosis (arrow) and no stenosis in the neck vessels. An antiplatelet agent was started. His neurological symptom gradually improved.

The stroke mechanism was an artery to artery embolization from the left distal ICA to the MCA pial zones.

• Case 12

A 50-year-old man was referred to our hospital for a further management. He had numbness of his right elbow 1 month before admission and had been treated with an antiplatelet agent. He also complained of right limb weakness, swallowing difficulty, and language disturbance since 1 week before. The symptoms occurred while typing and lasted for several hours. He had a history of untreated hypertension and hypercholesterolemia for 5 years, and he was a 60-pack-year current smoker. His heart rhythm was regular without murmur, and carotid bruit was inaudible. His spontaneous speech and naming was slightly impaired. He showed Gerstmann features and paraphasic errors. He showed a weakness (MRC grade IV) and hypesthesia in the right limbs. There were no abnormal findings in both transthoracic echocardiography and transesophageal echocardiography.

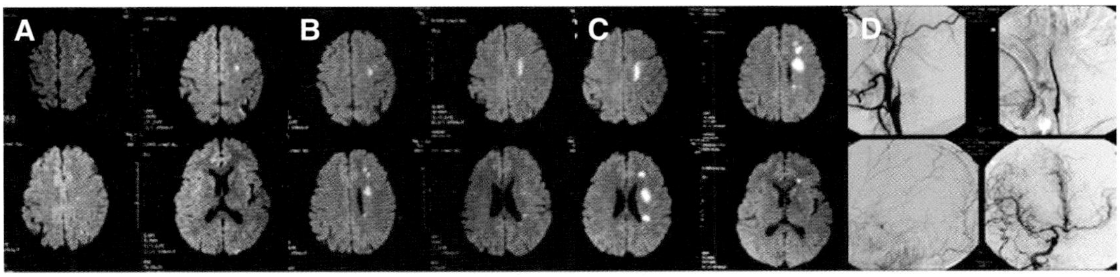

On Brain MR-DWI (A-C), multiple small ischemic lesions were noticed in the left basal ganglia, high frontal cortex, subcortex, and internal borderzone area (A: 1 month ago; B: 1 week ago; C: 2 days ago). On conventional angiography (D), the left intracavernous ICA was barely visualized through ophthalmic artery due to a distal occlusion. The left MCA was supplied by the right ACA through the Acom and the PCA through the Pcom. On brain SPECT, there was decreased perfusion and vascular reserve in the left MCA territory. He was managed with intravenous unfractionated heparin, because of recurrent ischemic attacks while taking antiplatelet medication. He did not experience any other symptoms thereafter, and the NIHSS improved from 6 to 3 at discharge.

The presumed stroke mechanism was recurrent artery to artery emboli from the distal ICA above the siphon, which migrated into the end-artery zones. He did not have any hemodynamic episodes, but an angiogram and SPECT showed decreased vascular reserve in the left MCA territory. Therefore, another possible mechanism was the progression of low flow infarctions, just like the extension of the lesions on the three DWIs over 1 month.

• Case 13

A 67-year-old right-handed man came to our hospital for right-sided weakness. He had a 10-year medical history of diabetes mellitus, a 3-year history of hypertension and a 1-year history of chronic renal failure. However, he had not experienced any stroke symptoms until he felt a sudden right-sided weakness while resting in the morning on the day of admission. He did not complain of mental change, dysarthria and aphasia. He had a right-sided weakness estimated as an MRC grade IV+, but the exam of the cranial nerves, sensory system and deep tendon reflexes were normal. Transthoracic echocardiography and Holter monitoring did not reveal any cardiac sources of embolism.

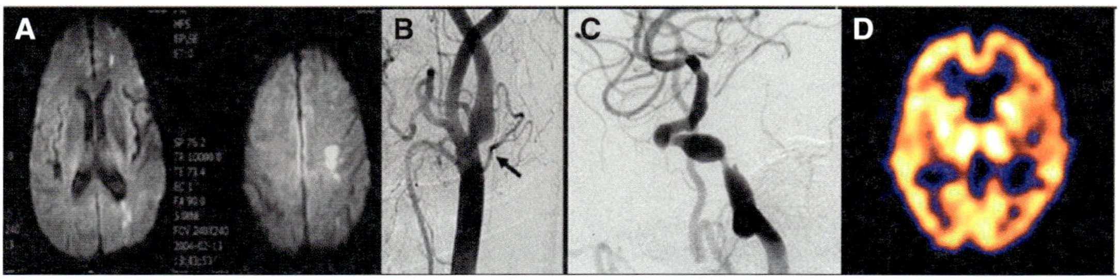

Brain MR-DWI (A) showed multifocal infarctions in the left frontoparietooccipital lobe. Conventional angiography (B, C) showed multiple stenoses in the left proximal and distal ICA. Brain SPECT (D) showed decreased perfusion and vascular reserve in left fronto-parietal lobe. He was treated with aspirin, and his limb weakness improved after 2 weeks of admission. We considered delayed intervention of the stenotic portion of the left ICA.

Although there was a decreased vascular reserve and borderzone lesions, the stroke mechanism was thought to be an artery to artery embolization from the proximal ICA stenosis or multiple distal ICA tandem lesions.

• Case 14

A 70-year-old man was admitted because of a left-sided weakness. History taking revealed that he had suffered from hypertension and diabetes mellitus for almost 10 years, for which he had taken regular medication. He had no history of heart disease or previous stroke. He was alert and oriented with intact cognitive functions. There was no motor or visual neglect on the left side. Cranial nerve examinations were normal except for mild dysarthria. His left extremities were mildly weak (MRC grade IV+). Sensory examination showed no abnormal findings. Ataxia, tremor and gait abnormality were not noted. ECG and echocardiography showed no remarkable abnormal findings.

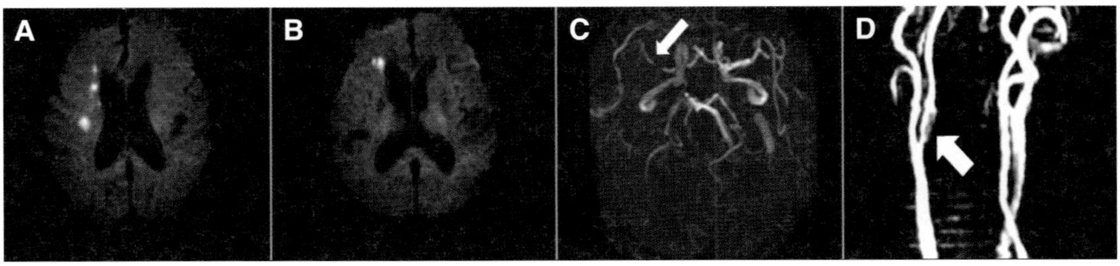

Brain MR-DWI (A, B) showed multiple punctate lesions in the right centrum semiovale. Brain MRA showed severe stenosis of the right M1 (C, arrow) and mild stenosis of the right proximal ICA (D, arrow). He was treated with dual antiplatelet agents. His neurological deficit improved completely.

The putative stroke mechanism was an artery to artery embolization from the stenotic MCA or proximal ICA to the perforator zone of the MCA.

• Case 15

A 65-year-old man presented with left hemiparesis. Suddenly, he felt a tingling sensation on his left arm and weakness of his left hand 1 day prior to visit. He had hypertension and a family history of stroke. He was a heavy smoker and alcoholic. On neurologic examination, there were no cortical symptoms and cranial nerve functions were normal. Motor power of the left upper extremity was MRC grade IV of the proximal and grade II of the distal limb. Sensory was mildly impaired for all modalities on the left arm. Deep tendon reflexes were normal. Transthoracic echocardiography and Holter monitoring did not reveal any cardiac sources of embolism.

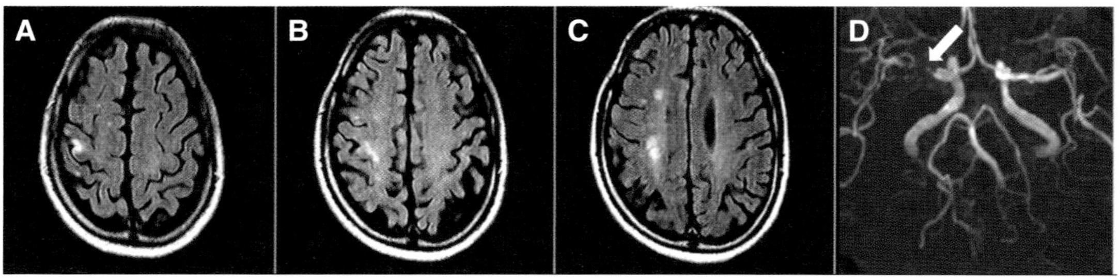

Brain MRI (A-C) showed multifocal acute infarctions in the right MCA territory. Brain MRA (D) showed a significant stenosis at the right M1 segment. He was treated with an antiplatelet agent.

The mechanism of stroke was thought to be an artery to artery embolism from the MCA stem embolizing to the distal branches. His symptoms sparing the lower extremities resulted from the topographical distribution of the affected motor cortex.

• Case 16

A 58-year-old man visited our hospital because of clumsiness of his right hand and a tingling sensation of his right upper extremity. He had a history of hypertension and smoking of 30 packyears. His mental status was intact. He had a right central type facial palsy. Other cranial nerves were normal. Motor power of the right side was MRC grade IV+. Sensory examination revealed no objective abnormalities. Echocardiography revealed atherosclerosis of the aortic arch.

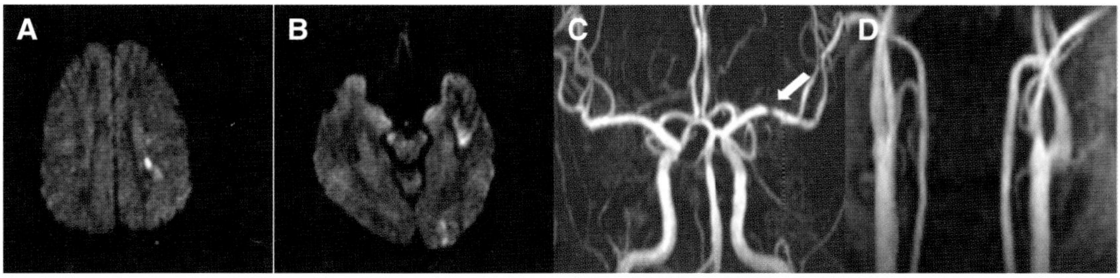

Brain MR-DWI (A, B) showed multiple acute infarctions in the left centrum semiovale, caudate nucleus head, occipital lobe and left anterior temporal lobe. Brain MRA showed focal stenosis at the mid portion of the left MCA stem (C) and intact proximal arteries (D).We started antiplatelet medication and his symptoms improved.

The stroke mechanism was an artery to artery embolism from the left MCA to the distal parts.

• Case 17

A 79-year-old man visited our hospital complaining of a sudden left-sided weakness and dysarthria. 2 years before, he had been diagnosed with multiple bilateral hemispheric infarcts and had been admitted to an outside hospital and treated with warfarin and aspirin. He had a history of hypertension, heart disease and diabetes mellitus. Upon visiting the emergency room, his BP was 150/90mmHg. His mental state was alert and oriented. Cranial nerve examination showed a central type left facial palsy, dysarthria and dysphagia. There was a left-sided (MRC grade II) and right-sided weakness (MRC grade IV+, previous stroke sequelae). Deep tendon reflexes were brisk and Babinski sign was positive on the left. Serum laboratory results, ECG, and transthoracic echocardiography were all normal.

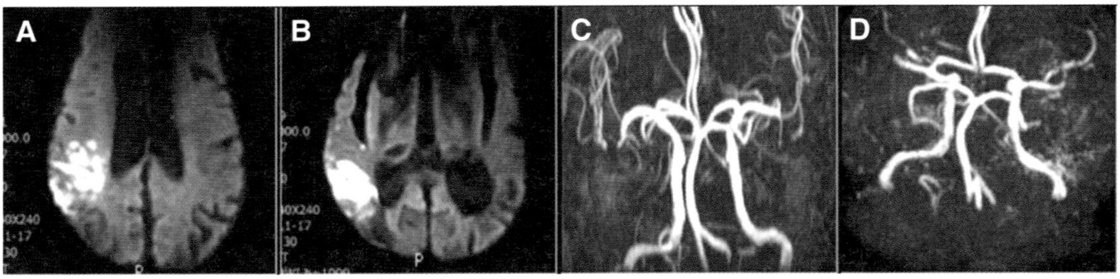

Brain MR-DWI (A, B) showed an acute infarct in the right posterior temporoparietal lobe. An MRA performed 3 years before revealed a focal stenosis of the right MCA (C). However, a brain MRA at performed during the current visit showed an occlusion of the inferior division of the right MCA (D). Extracranial vessels were intact. The patient was diagnosed with an infiltrating adenocarcinoma on a colonoscopy after his admission. He was treated with clopidogrel and discharged without improvement.

The mechanism of stroke was thought to be an artery to artery embolic infarct from the stenotic MCA to the inferior division.

• Case 18

A 64-year-old man was hospitalized because of weakness of his right leg and dysarthria, which had occurred 11 days before admission. He had a history of hypertensive intracerebral hemorrhage of the left parietal area 10 years ago. 7 months ago, he had felt weakness and hypesthesia of the left side, and had been diagnosed with an acute infarction of the right MCA territory. Thereafter, he had taken aspirin. 2 months ago, he had been diagnosed with pancreatic cancer and was on chemotherapy. His mental status was intact. He had dysarthria and weakness of his right leg. Sensation over the face and body was intact. Cerebellar function test revealed terminal dysmetria of the left limbs. Echocardiography showed no abnormal findings.

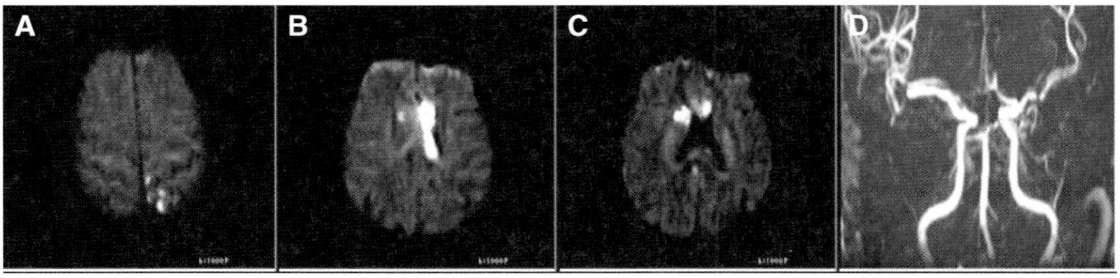

Brain MR-DWI (A-C) showed acute multifocal infarctions in the left ACA territories and the right basal ganglia. Brain MRA (D) showed significant stenoses of the left distal M1 and both ACAs. On TCD, moderate stenoses of the MCA, VA and ACA were noted. Antiplatelet agent was changed from aspirin to clopidogrel. His symptoms improved slightly.

The basal ganglia was thought to be supplied by the recurrent artery of Heubner possibly originating from the Acom or left ACA. The stroke mechanism might be an artery to artery embolism from the left ACA to both ACA territories.

• Case 19

A 66-year-old man came to our hospital with recurrent left lower extremity weakness. He had a history of hypertension and a right thalamic infarction 4 years ago, for which he was treated with antihypertensive medication and aspirin. 6 days prior to admission, he had felt a sudden weakness of his left lower extremity, which had resolved after 5 minutes. He experienced the same symptoms twice a day until admission. His neurologic examination was normal. Echocardiography and Holter monitoring did not reveal any specific abnormalities.

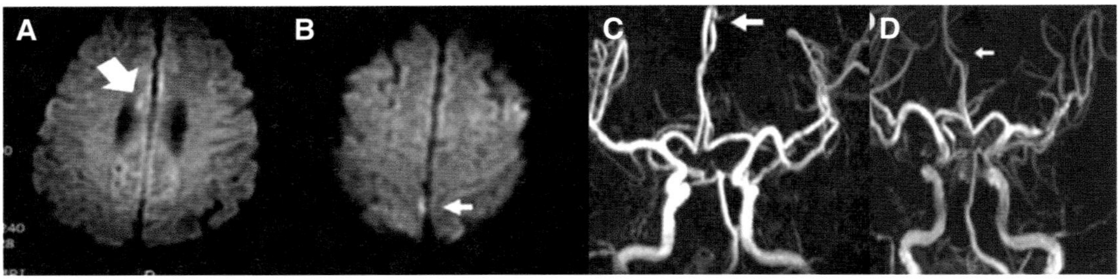

Brain MR-DWI (A, B) showed small acute infarctions in the body of the right corpus callosum and cortex of the right parietal lobe (arrows). Brain MRA (C, D) showed severe stenosis of the right distal ACA (arrows). He had taken aspirin since the previous thalamic infarction, and his treatment was changed to dual antiplatelet agents due to recurrent strokes.

His stroke was thought to be due to an artery to artery embolization from the stenotic right ACA. The clinical diagnosis is a TIA, and the TIA mechanism is embolic in this case.

• Case 20

A 69-year-old woman who had a 10-year history of hypertension presented with dizziness and altered mentality. 2 weeks before admission, she had been treated with a combination of aspirin and clopidogrel due to an acute infarction of the left cerebellum at an outside hospital. But, no neurologic deficit remained. On the day of admission, dizziness and altered mentality developed during dish washing. She became comatose. Light reflexes were prompt and doll's eye test was intact. All four extremities were flaccid. Deep tendon reflexes were hyperactive on the left side. Echocardiographic examination showed no abnormal findings.

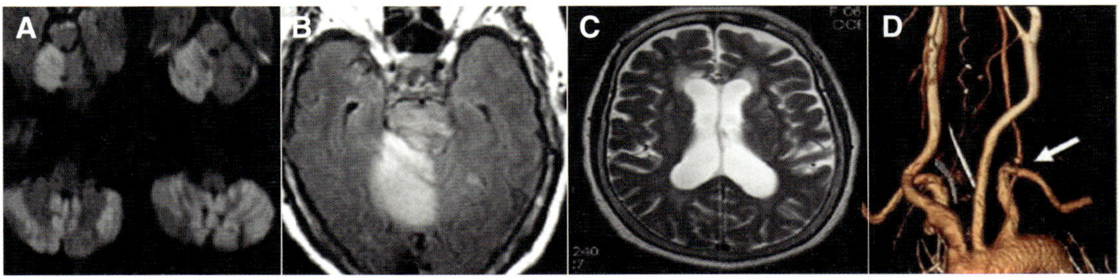

Brain MR-DWI (A) revealed bilateral cerebellar infarctions. The initial NIHSS was 40 and intravenous rt-PA was administered. Her mental state improved to a drowsy state, but 2 days later, she became comatose again. A follow-up MRI (B) showed a mass effect compressing the brainstem due to the massive acute infarction in the bilateral cerebellar hemispheres and new infarctions in the pons. T2WI image (C) showed mild hydrocephalus secondary to the extensive cerebellar lesions. CT angiography (D) revealed a focal stenosis of the left VA orifice, and a diffuse stenosis of the right VA. Because of the development of a new stroke while on an antiplatelet combination, she was treated with anticoagulation.

Recurrent infarctions developed during the first 2 days. Because there was no severe hydrocephalus, the aggravation of the mental state was likely due to the new infarction in the pons. The stroke mechanism was an artery to artery embolization from the severe stenotic portion of the left proximal VA or the right VA.

• Case 21

A 66-year-old man presented with sudden dizziness and episodes of vertical diplopia. His medical history included rectal cancer treated with Miles' operation 14 years ago, but no vascular risk factors. His symptoms had continued to fluctuate for several weeks. At the emergency room, he was drowsy. Neurologic examination revealed vertical diplopia and partial gaze limitation with gaze-evoked nystagmus. He had a right facial palsy of central origin and mild dysarthria. Mild hypesthesia was detected on the left face. He showed right arm dysmetria. Transthoracic echocardiography and Holter monitoring did not reveal any cardiac sources of embolism.

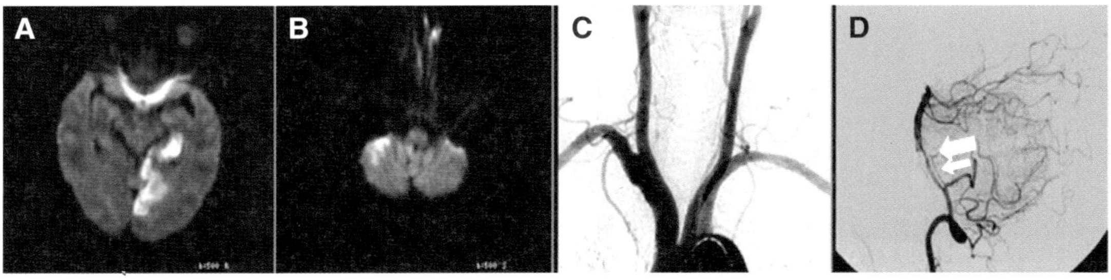

We treated him with heparin due to his recurrent posterior TIAs. In spite of anticoagulation treatment, right upper limb hemiparesis and right side homonymous hemianopsia developed. Brain MR-DWI showed acute infarctions in the left PCA (A) and bilateral PICA territories (B). Conventional angiography showed right proximal VA occlusion (C) and left distal VA stenosis (D). TCD revealed increased flow velocities of the left VA and BA. No further attacks occurred thereafter.

The emboli could have originated from the right VA considering the right cerebellar lesion and the left occipital lesion. However, TFCA showed that the right VA was occluded at a proximal site and the left distal VA was stenotic. Also, both PICA territories were supplied by the left PICA on conventional angiography. The stroke mechanism was an artery to artery embolism from the left distal VA. Because of his fluctuating symptoms, we decided to treat him with short term oral anticoagulation followed by an antiplatelet.

• Case 22

A 63-year-old man with altered mentality visited the emergency room. He was drowsy and vomiting. He had a previous left basal ganglia hemorrhage 7 years ago. Also he had diabetes mellitus and hypertension. His brain stem reflexes were all intact. His right limbs were weak (MRC grade III) and his left limbs were weaker (MRC grade I). Left-sided hypesthesia and upper motor neuron signs were noticed. Serial ECG and Holter monitoring could not detect atrial fibrillation. There was no significant finding except a low ejection fraction on transthoracic echocardiography and transesophageal echocardiography.

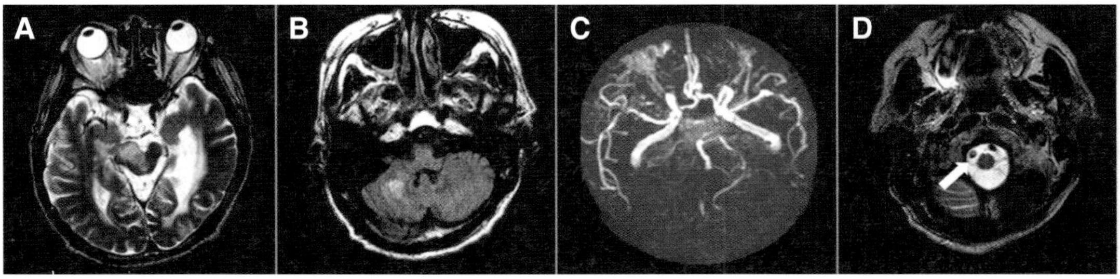

Brain MRI (A, B) showed an acute ischemic infarction in the right brain stem and right cerebellum. Brain MRA (C) showed no visible right VA and poor visualization of the right PCA. T2WI (D, arrow) showed an irregular lumen of the right VA. He was treated with anticoagulation. His mentality and weakness improved slightly. However, he had recurrent angina pectoris.

There was a T2 high signal intensity lesion in the lumen of the right VA on brain MRI, and multiple infarcts in the posterior circulation were confirmed. So, the stroke mechanism may have been an artery to artery embolism from the right VA to more distal arteries. We can see the thrombus within vascular signal void in the right basilar top, proximal PCA and VA on the T2WI.

• Case 23

An 82-year-old man presented with vertigo. He had a 10-year history of hypertension and diabetes mellitus. 14 hours before visiting hospital, he felt dizzy and complained of vertigo while resting in bed. His vertigo developed intermittently for several seconds without relation to position. But the dizziness persisted and was accompanied by nausea and vomiting. He was alert. There was no nystagmus, hemiparesis and sensory change. Cerebellar function test including finger to finger, finger to nose and heel to shin tests were all intact. But he couldn't walk due to his dizziness. Transthoracic echocardiography and Holter monitoring did not reveal any cardiac sources of embolism.

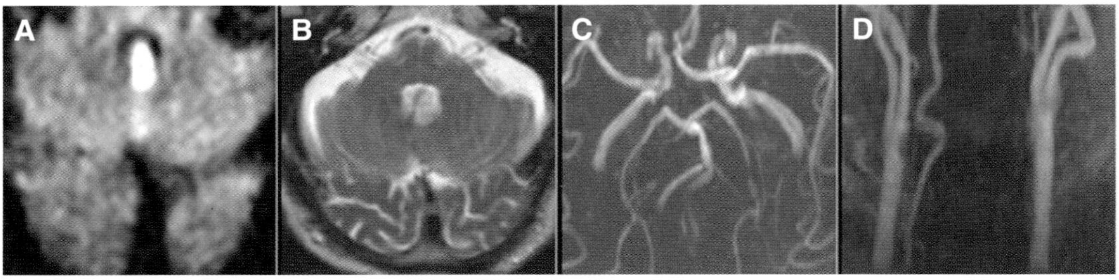

Brain MRI (A, B) showed an acute infarction of the left cerebellar vermis and uvula. Brain MRA (C, D) showed diffuse stenosis of the left vertebral artery. Antiplatelet was prescribed. His dizziness completely improved at discharge.

The stroke mechanism was an artery to artery embolization from the left VA to the medial PICA. A PICA territory infarction should differentiate in isolated vertigo mimicking labyrinthitis. Vertigo can be explained by involvement of the uvulonodular complex of the vermis, which is part of the vestibular portion of the cerebellum.[8]

• Case 24

A 61-year-old woman visited the emergency department complaining of dizziness and dysphagia. She had a history of hypertension and diabetes mellitus. Dizziness and dysphagia developed suddenly 4 hours prior to admission during dinner. Motor weakness and hypesthesia were absent. She showed a left veering tendency. On neurologic examination, her mental state was clear and cranial examination revealed no abnormalities except dysphagia. Motor power was normal and the sensory system was intact. On the cerebellar function test, there was a left-sided ataxia. Transthoracic echocardiography and Holter monitoring did not reveal any cardiac sources of embolism.

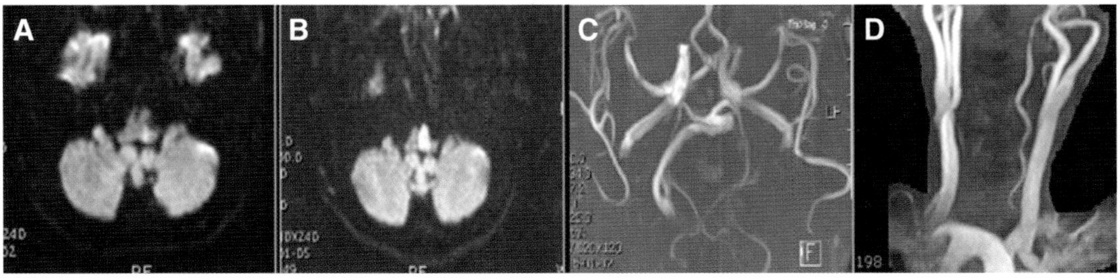

Brain MR-DWI (A) showed acute infarctions in the medial portion of the left lateral medulla. After 3 days, a new acute infarction in the left medial medulla was detected (B). On brain MRA (C, D), the left VA was hypoplastic. Initially we treated the patient with aspirin and clopidogrel. Because she presented with recurrent weakness, we started intravenous anticoagulation. Her symptoms improved gradually.

Both lateral and medial medullary infarctions are rare. About 3% of patients with medullary infarctions presented with both lateral and medial medullary infarctions.[9] The mechanism of ischemic stroke in this patient was thought to be an artery to artery embolism from the stenotic, hypoplastic left VA.

• Case 25

A 56-year-old man presented with dysarthria and dizziness that developed 6 days before admission. His medical history included hypertension with regular treatment for 6 years. He was a current smoker of 30 packyears. He was alert. His neurologic examination was unremarkable except for left limb at axia. Carotid and ophthalmic bruits were inaudible. Echocardiographic examination was normal.

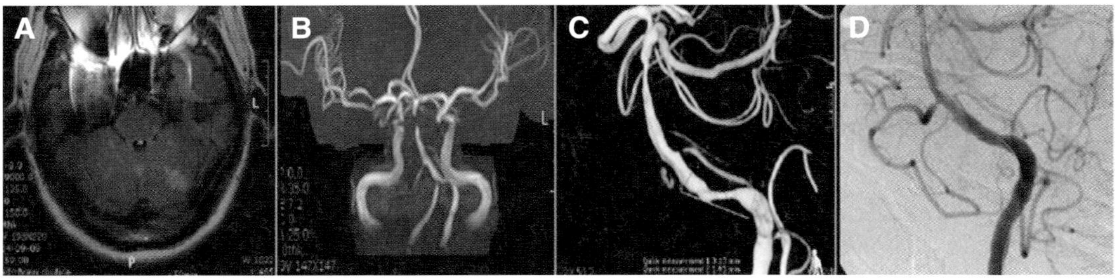

Brain MRI (A) showed a left cerebellar infarction. Brain MRA (B) and conventional angiography (C) showed a focal stenosis of both distal VAs and mid-BA. Initially, anticoagulation was administered to this patient. Stenting in BA and left distal VA was performed (D). There were no complications and no further attacks.

The vascular territory of the cerebellar lesion is not definite for the SCA or PICA. But the angiographic studies showed that the BA was more stenotic than the VA. Thus, an embolism from mid-BA to the SCA territory is a more plausible scenario. Stenting of BA and VA in this patient is controversial. The interventional procedure can be reserved for a second ischemic event despite best medical treatment.

• Case 26

A 64-year-old woman visited the ER with sudden vertigo, vomiting and dysarthria. Her past medical history revealed hypertension and diabetes mellitus, and she had undergone radiotherapy due to cervical cancer 15 years before. Her neurologic examination revealed dysarthria and limb ataxia of the left side. Abnormal findings were not observed on laboratory tests. Echocardiography was normal.

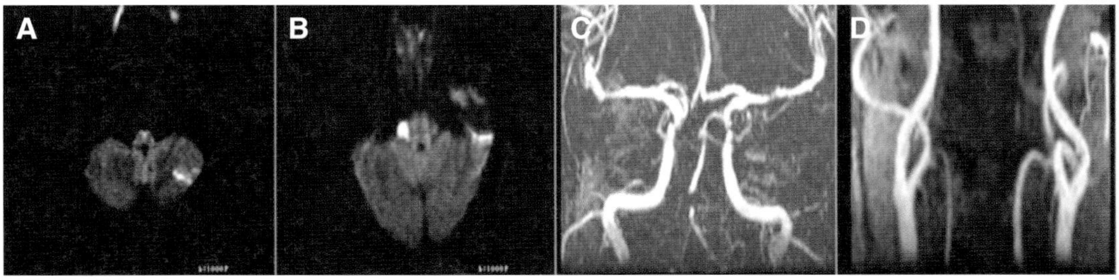

Brain MR-DWI (A, B) showed acute infarcts in the right pons and the left AICA territory. Brain MRA revealed multifocal stenoses in the proximal BA, both distal ICAs, and left MCA (C). Extracranial arteries were intact (D). She was treated with dual antiplatelet agents, and her symptoms improved.

Her stroke may be due to an artery to artery embolization from the BA to the left AICA territory and the right pons (and possibly the right AICA territory).

• Case 27

A 58-year-old man with visual disturbance and dizziness visited the emergency room. He had a previous right lateral medullary infarction, which had been diagnosed 7 years before. He was taking aspirin for secondary stroke prevention. Also he had diabetes mellitus and hypertension. He was alert. His brain stem reflexes were all intact. Visual field exam revealed a left superior quadrantanopsia. Motor and sensory examinations of all extremities were normal. Serial ECGs and Holter monitoring did not detect atrial fibrillation. There was no significant finding on transthoracic echocardiography and transesophageal echocardiography.

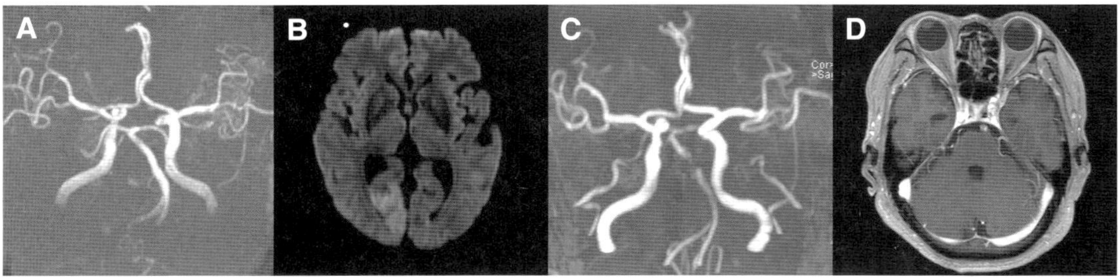

Brain MRA, which had been performed 7 years before (A), showed a suspicious basilar stenotic lesion. Brain MR-DWI taken during the current admission (B) showed acute ischemic infarctions in both PCA territories, and brain MRA (C) revealed a severe stenosis of mid-BA. T1 enhanced image (D) showed an irregular lumen of BA. He was treated with dual antiplatelet agents.

There was an atheroma in the lumen of the BA on brain MRA, and multiple infarcts in the posterior circulation were confirmed. The stroke mechanism may be artery to artery embolisms from the BA to more distal arteries. There had been progressive intracranial atherosclerosis in the BA, which might have ruptured recently. This can be confirmed with recent imaging techniques such as plaque imaging of the BA, by comparing the plaque images between the attack and images taken 3 months later.

• Case 28

A 60-year-old man visited hospital complaining of left visual blurring that had developed 3 days before. The duration of visual blurring was within a few minutes, and the symptom recovered spontaneously. There was no motor or sensory change. He had a history of hypertension, diabetes mellitus, and dyslipidemia. Upon visiting the emergency room, his BP was 160/90mmHg. He was alert and oriented. His neurologic examination revealed no remarkable findings except for a bruit over the left neck. Serum laboratory results, ECG, and transthoracic echocardiography were all normal.

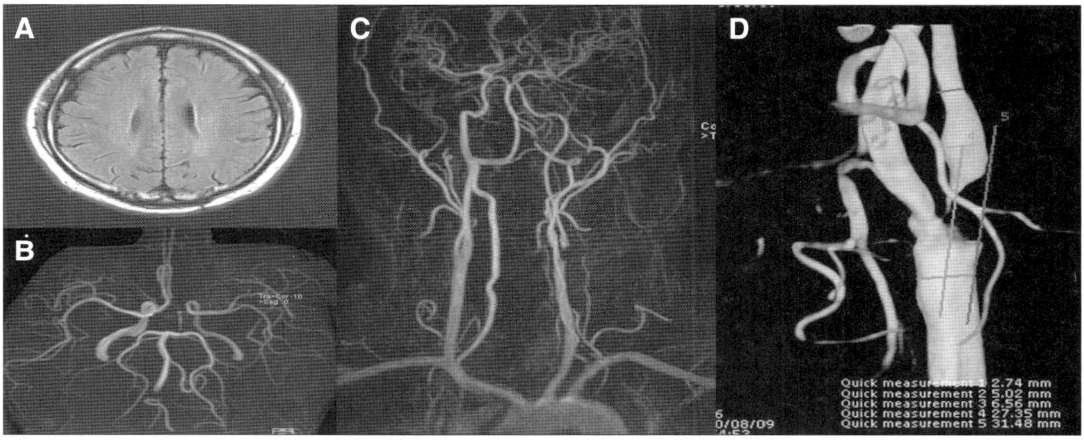

Brain MRI (A) showed no acute or subacute infarct in the left hemisphere. The signal intensity was decreased in the left ICA and MCA on TOF-MRA (B). Contrast neck MRA showed a severe stenosis of the left proximal ICA (C, D). The patient was diagnosed with transient monocular blindness associated with an unstable left proximal ICA atherosclerotic lesion and endartectomy was performed. He was prescribed aspirin and clopidogrel. He had no further attacks thereafter.

The mechanism of stroke was thought to be an artery to artery embolic infarct from the unstable left proximal ICA atherosclerotic lesion to the ophthalmic artery.

• Case 29

A 45-year-old man visited the emergency room. On awaking in the morning, he had left limb weakness and dysarthria. He was a 20-pack-year current smoker, but did not have any other stroke risk factors. He had fallen down from a train 30 years before and had been treated surgically with no neurologic sequelae. His heart beat was regular without murmur. Carotid bruit was inaudible. There was a mild left limb weakness (MRC grade IV) and vibratory hypesthesia. All laboratory findings were within normal limits. Transthoracic echocardiography did not reveal any abnormal findings.

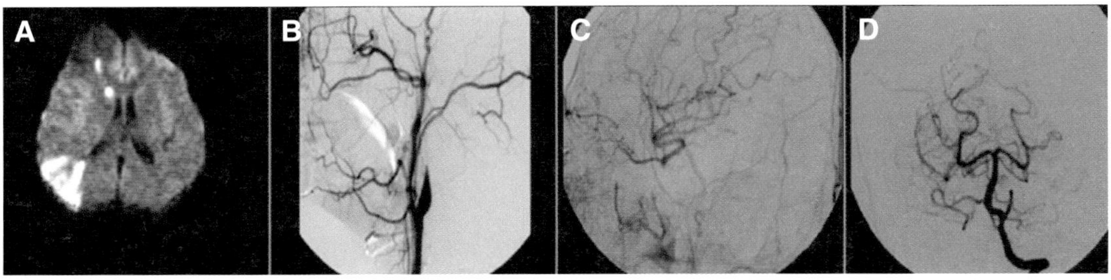

There were multiple acute infarctions in the right parietal lobe, anterior frontal subcortex, and basal ganglia on brain MR-DWI (A). Conventional angiography (B-D) revealed an occlusion of the right proximal ICA. Furthermore, the right MCA flow was faintly visualized through the OA and Pcom. At first, he was treated with dual antiplatelet agents, clopidogrel and aspirin. However, he came to our hospital again 4 months later, because he had a sudden, brief visual loss of the right eye that lasted 1 minute. His medication was changed to warfarin thereafter.

The flow to the right ophthalmic artery and posterior communicating artery was supplied by the right MCA. The ischemic lesion was mainly located in the territory of the right posterior parietal artery coexisting with several small anterior frontal and basal ganglia lesions. Although the vascular reserve of the right MCA territory was decreased, the most reasonable stroke mechanism was thought to be an artery to artery embolization from the distal stump of the proximal ICA occlusion site by reversed ophthalmic flow. His occasional amaurosis fugax could be explained by embolization from the proximal stump of the ICA occlusion via the ECA through the ophthalmic artery. Warfarin was administered in this patient for the inhibition of new thrombus formations around the proximal stump. In addition, the surgical anastomosis of the right superficial temporal artery and MCA could be another choice of treatment later.

1-2. In situ thrombosis

• Case 30

An 84-year-old woman was referred to the emergency room because of a sudden left-sided weakness. 3 days prior to her visit, her left limb became suddenly weak. 15 years before, she had been diagnosed with a left MCA infarction that caused a right-sided weakness. But she had been able to do daily life activities independently until prior to admission. She was not taking medication for the secondary prevention of stroke. She had no other stroke risk factors. She was alert and dysarthric. There was no hemi-neglect. Limb and facial weakness on the left side was detected. Sensory examination revealed no abnormal findings. ECG and transthoracic echocardiography showed no significant findings.

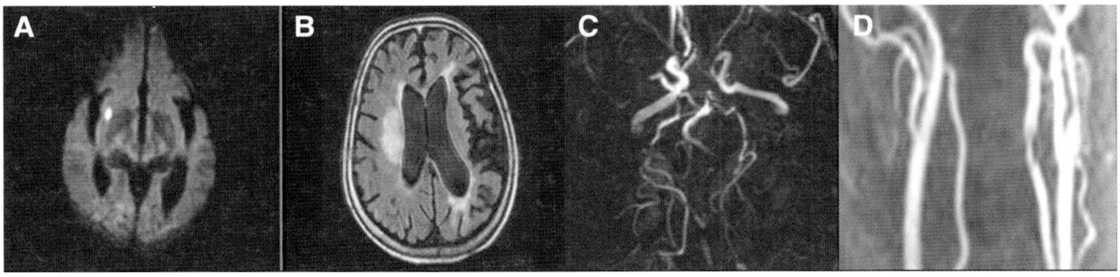

Brain MR-DWI (A) showed an acute infarction in the right corona radiata and external capsule. A right striatocapsular infarction and cerebromalacia possibly due to an old infarction of the left MCA territory were detected on FLAIR imaging (B). Brain MRA (C, D) showed non-visualization of both MCAs and focal stenoses of both PCAs, left proximal ICA, and left mid VA. She was treated with an antiplatelet agent. Her neurological deficits were stationary.

There were diffuse atherosclerotic changes on brain MRA. No embolic sources were detected. The acute ischemic lesion involved the territory supplied by MCA perforators. Thus, the stroke mechanism was thought to be an in situ thrombosis of the right MCA stem.

• Case 31

A 55-year-old man visited the emergency room because of right-sided weakness that developed 7 days before admission. At that time, she slipped down and developed a right hip fracture. She did not have dysarthria, dysphagia or other symptoms. She had a past medical history of hypertension, hypercholesterolemia, angina and diabetes mellitus. She was alert and oriented. Cranial nerve examinations showed no abnormal findings. Her motor power of her right upper extremity was MRC grade III+, but her right lower extremity was not checkable due to her immediate post-op state. Echocardiography showed no abnormal findings.

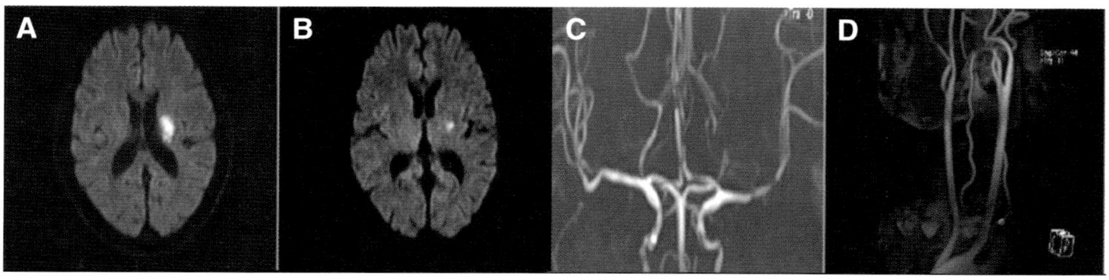

Brain MR-DWI (A, B) showed acute ischemic infarctions in the left corona radiata and internal capsule. Brain MRA (C, D) showed multifocal narrowing of the left MCA M1 segment and left proximal PCA. Mild narrowing of both distal cavernous ICAs and distal petrous portions were suspected. We started her on antiplatelet agent medication.

The stroke mechanism of this patient might be an in situ thrombosis of the left MCA. However, the diagnosis of small vessel occlusion (lacune) due to branch atheromatose disease is possible.

• Case 32

A 62-year-old right-handed man presented with a sudden left-sided weakness on the day of his visit. He had suffered from hypertension for 10 years and was on regular medication. He was alert and oriented. Cranial nerve examination showed a left central type facial palsy and dysarthria. Motor power of the left limb was MRC grade IV-. Sensory function was intact. Echocardiogram showed no remarkable findings except for concentric LVH.

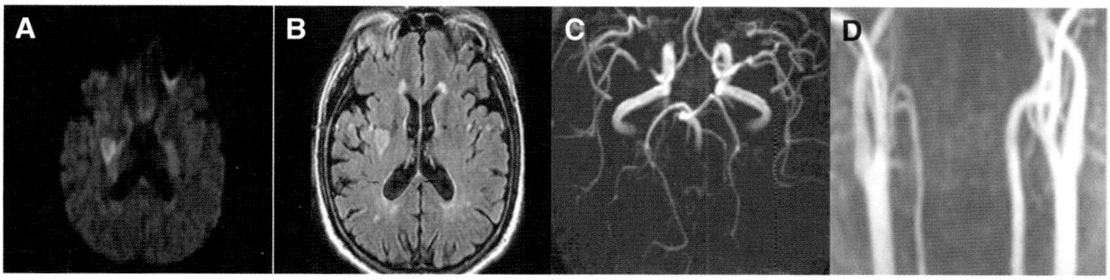

Brain MRI (A, B) showed an acute infarction in the MCA perforator zone. Brain MRA (C, D) showed a severe right MCA stenosis and no remarkable findings in the neck vessels. He was treated initially with aspirin. However, the treatment was changed into anticoagulation because of the progression of his weakness.

Embolic sources were not detected in the heart and proximal ICAs. The stroke mechanism was an in situ thrombosis of the right MCA stem. In this case, the treatment was changed to anticoagulation because of symptom progression. However, the use of anticoagulation in stroke in evolution is a controversial subject in the treatment of stroke.

• Case 33

A 59-year-old left-handed woman presented with a sudden onset of headache and left arm tingling sensation. Her medical history included diabetes mellitus diagnosed 10 years ago. She was alexic without agraphia. Cranial nerve examination showed no abnormal findings except for a left homonymous hemianopsia. Motor power, sensory and cerebellar functions were all normal. Echocardiographic findings did not reveal any abnormal findings.

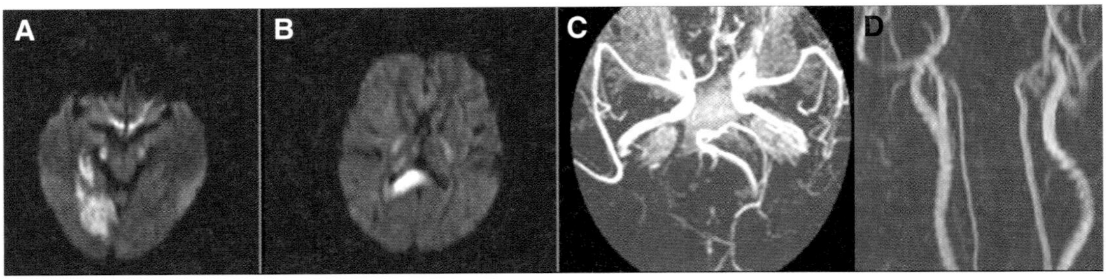

Brain MR-DWI (A, B) showed high signal intensity lesions in the right occipital lobe, thalamus, and splenium. Brain MRA (C, D) showed a diffuse narrowing of the right PCA and no other remarkable findings. He was treated with aspirin, and his symptoms were stationary throughout his admission.

The patient had alexia without agraphia, one of the disconnection signs. Her speech center might be located in the right hemisphere. The stroke mechanism was thought be an in situ thrombosis of the right PCA.

• Case 34

A 70-year-old man visited our hospital due to sudden dysarthria and right-sided weakness. He had a past medical history of diabetes mellitus, hypertension and Parkinson's disease. 4 hours before admission, he felt weak on the right side and dysarthria after bathing. His neurologic examination revealed dysarthria and right-sided weakness (MRC grade IV). His sensory examination was normal. ECG and echocardiography were all normal.

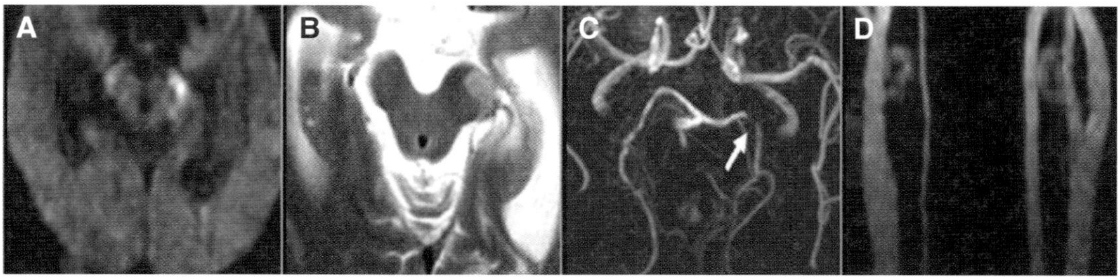

Brain MRI (A, B) showed an acute ischemic infarction in the cerebral peduncle of the left midbrain. Brain MRA (C, D) revealed a focal stenosis of the left proximal PCA. He was treated with an anticoagulant. However, at the third admission day, the right-sided weakness progressed to MRC grade II.

The most common site of atherosclerotic stenosis of the PCA is its winding portion around midbrain.[10] There was no embolic source in the proximal VA and heart. The stroke mechanism was thought to be an in situ thrombosis of the left PCA.

• Case 35

A 68-year-old man was admitted because of a sudden right-sided weakness and ipsilateral hemibody tingling sensation. He had suffered from hypertension as was taking medication irregularly. He had no history of diabetes mellitus, heart disease or previous stroke. He was alert, but disoriented to time and place. Language functions were intact. Cranial nerve examinations revealed mild dysarthria. His right extremities were mildly weak (MRC grade IV+). Sensory examination showed right side sensory loss to all modalities. ECG and echocardiography showed no remarkable abnormalities.

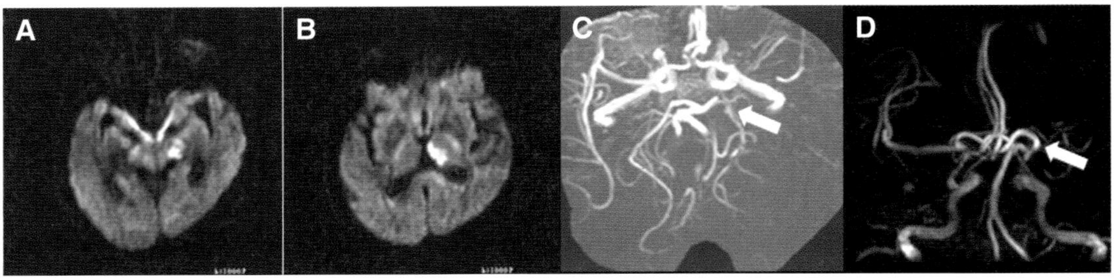

Brain MR-DWI (A, B) showed 2 discrete acute infarctions in the left medial midbrain and in the left medial thalamus. Brain MRA (C, D) showed severe stenosis in the left proximal PCA and left MCA. He was treated with an antiplatelet agent. His neurological symptoms improved gradually.

The stroke mechanism was thought to be an in situ thrombosis. However, the possibility of an artery to artery embolism from the proximal artery to the PCA cannot be excluded.

• Case 36

An 81-year-old woman presented with sudden vertigo on the day of her visit. This was accompanied by dysarthria and dysphagia. Her medical history included hypertension and diabetes mellitus under regular treatment. Her mental status was alert. Cranial nerve examinations showed dysarthria, dysphagia and a soft palate elevation limitation on the left side. Her facial motor and sensory functions were normal. Motor power was normal. Sensory examination revealed 50% hypesthesia of the right extremities. Cerebellar function tests showed dysmetria on the left side. ECG and echocardiographic examinations were all normal.

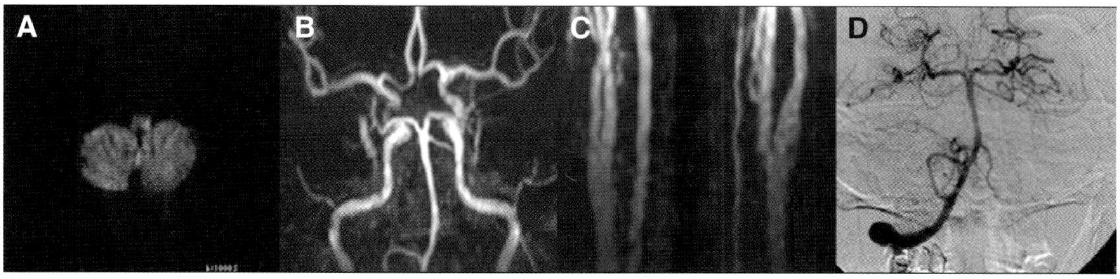

Brain MR-DWI (A) showed an acute infarction in the left lateral medulla. Brain MRA (B, C) showed hypoplasia of the left VA. Delayed dye washing of the left VA was noted during right vertebral angiography (D). An antiplatelet agent was started, and there was no neurological improvement. Aspiration pneumonia developed in this patient and progressed to acute respiratory distress syndrome. Finally, the patient expired due to infection.

The most common pathomechanism of lateral medullary infarction is an in situ thrombosis of the left VA as in this case.

• Case 37

4 days before admission, an 80-year-old man developed a gait disturbance and veering tendency to the left side. He also complained of headache, dizziness and dysarthria. He had hypertension and a history of right thalamic intracerebral hemorrhage (6 years ago). 3 years before, he had had a weakness of the left side, and taken herb medicine without visiting a doctor. His mentality was intact and alert. Cranial nerve examination revealed a left facial palsy and dysarthria. His motor power of the left side was MRC grade IV due to an old hemorrhagic stroke, but his sensory examination revealed no abnormal findings. He had severe limb ataxia and dysdiadochokinesia of the left side compared with the degree of weakness. Echocardiography revealed no abnormal findings.

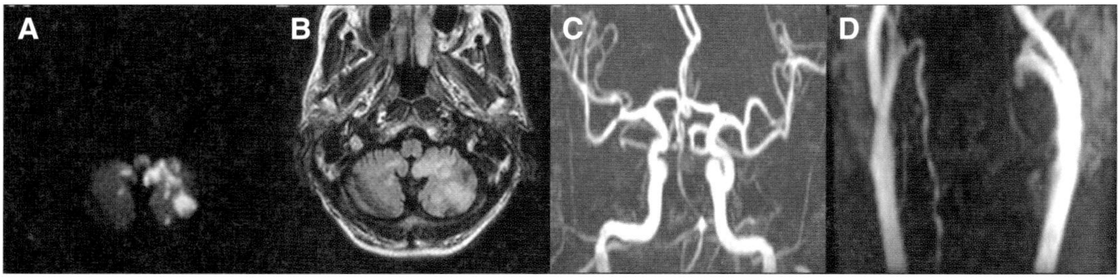

Brain MRI (A, B) showed acute infarctions in both cerebelli. Brain MRA showed diffuse narrowing of the BA (C) and no visualization of the left VA (D). We started the patient on anticoagulation, immediately. He could walk without aid at discharge.

The mechanism of stroke might be an in situ thrombosis of the left VA. Unilateral supply to both PICA territories is not rare.[11] The lesion in the right medial PICA territory was thought to be supplied by left PICA, and the spared areas were thought to be covered by the collaterals of the AICA and SCA. In patients with bilateral PICA infarctions, two topographic patterns of bilateral medial PICA or unilateral whole plus contralateral medial PICA involvement are frequently observed.[12] Most cases have unilateral PICA or unilateral vertebral artery disease. Thus, unilateral supply to both medial PICA territories may be the most relevant pathogenesis of this syndrome.

• Case 38

A 78-year-old woman was admitted to the emergency department because of a sudden dizziness and gait imbalance while walking. She had a history of hypertension and hypercholesterolemia. Her neurologic examination revealed bilateral limb dysmetria and a veering tendency. Visual perception of both eyes was normal. Other cranial nerve functions were normal. Strength, sensory perception, and deep tendon reflexes of all extremities were normal. Transthoracic echocardiography and Holter monitoring did not reveal any cardiac sources of embolism.

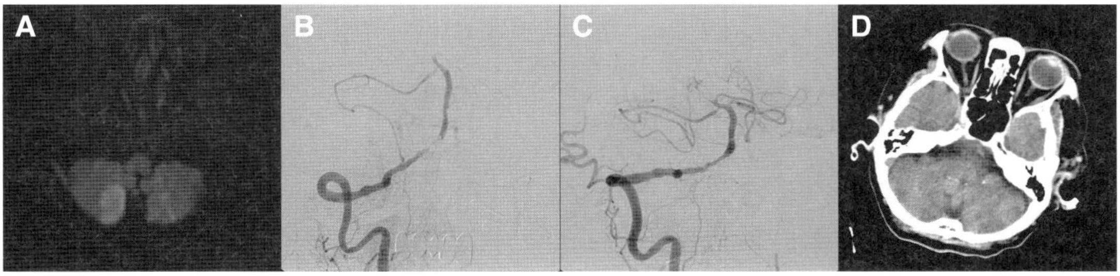

Brain MR-DWI (A) showed acute infarctions in both PICA territories. Conventional angiography (B) showed a severe stenosis of the right distal VA and hypoplasia of the left VA. She successfully underwent balloon angioplasty of the right distal VA (C). Brain CT 3 days after the angioplasty showed no evidence of brainstem infarcts, compression, or hydrocephalus (D). She improved completely and was discharged without further complications.

This patient had a dominant VA, which was severely stenotic. Emergent angioplasty prevented stroke progression. However, the long-term outcome of intracranial angioplasty remains unclear.

• Case 39

1 day ago, a 58-year-old man presented with headache and gait disturbance upon waking. He felt vertiginous with nausea and vomit. There were no motor and sensory symptoms. His medical history included hypertension and diabetes mellitus. His mental status was alert. Cranial nerve examinations and motor and sensory examinations showed no abnormalities. He showed left dysmetria on cerebellar function tests. Carotid or ophthalmic bruits were inaudible. FBS and HbA1c were 250mg/dL and 11.5%, respectively. Echocardiography showed no remarkable findings.

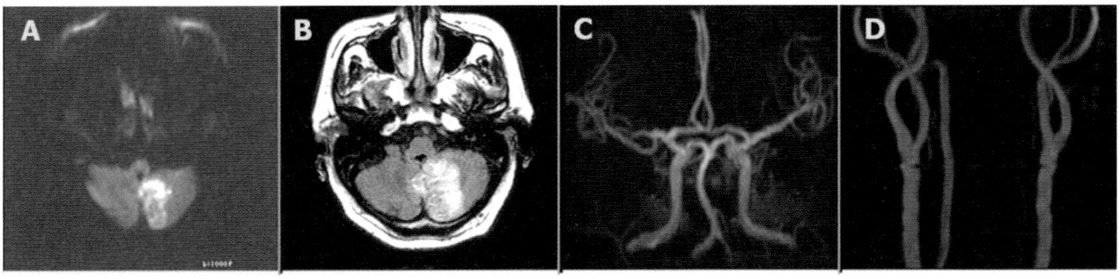

Brain MR-DWI (A, B) showed an acute infarction in the left PICA territory. Brain MRA (C, D) showed hypoplasia of the left VA. Aspirin and cilostazol were prescribed. He improved and was discharged.

The stroke mechanism was due to the left VA occlusion at the origin of the PICA.

• Case 40

A 67-year-old man presented with recurrent episodes of dysarthria and diplopia. He had a medical history of hypertension. 6 days prior to visiting the hospital, he had felt a sudden right-sided weakness, diplopia and dysarthria while bathing which lasted for 30 minutes. He had felt similar symptoms several times thereafter. 2 days later, he visited a local hospital, where thrombolysis was performed. However, the recurrent episodes persisted, and he visited our hospital for further treatment. Neurologic examination revealed a right-sided weakness (MRC grade IV+) and right-sided dysmetria. Intermittent drowsiness and limitation of right eye abduction were also seen. ECG and echocardiography were all normal.

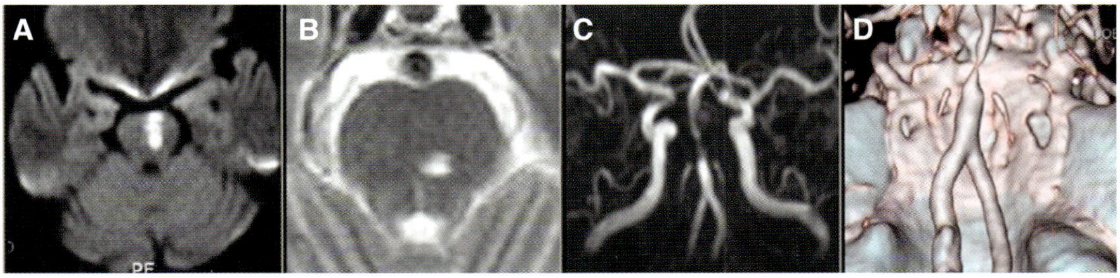

Brain MR-DWI (A) showed left medial pontine infarction. T2WI (B) showed an irregular lumen of the BA. Brain MRA (C) and CT angiography (D) revealed severe BA stenosis. He was treated with anticoagulation, but during anticoagulation, he experienced several attacks of drowsiness and right eye abduction limitation. Recurrent attacks subsided afterward, and he was discharged with warfarin.

The stroke mechanism was thought to be an in situ thrombosis of the stenotic portion of the BA. In contrast to usual lacunar infarctions, in situ thrombosis of the parent artery in these infarctions usually start from the most basal portion of the pons or MCA stem, although it is not a conclusive radiologic point.

• Case 41

A 50-year-old woman was admitted due to a sudden binocular diplopia. She had no definite motor or sensory symptoms. She had suffered from longstanding hypertension for 15 years. Neurologic examination showed an internuclear ophthalmoplegia. There were no abnormalities on motor or sensory examinations. ECG and echocardiographic examinations were all normal.

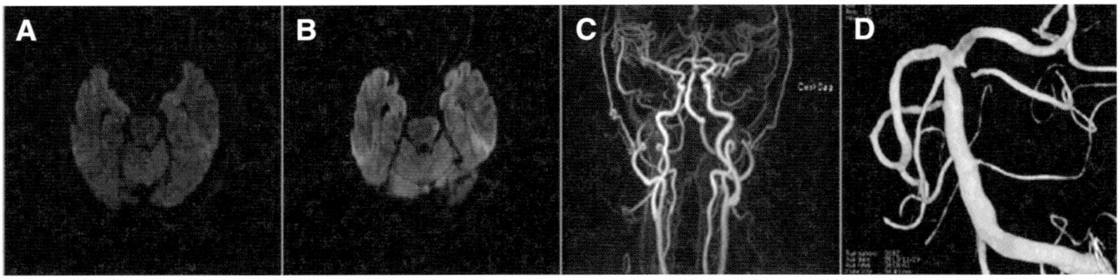

Brain MR-DWI (A, B) showed an acute infarction involving the territory of the long circumferential artery territory. Brain MRA (C) showed a moderate stenosis of the distal BA. Conventional angiography (D) showed a moderate stenosis of the BA and severe stenosis of the SCA. The long circumferential artery on the left was not noted on TFCA. She had progressive weakness of the right arm over 1 day. The extent of the infarction increased. She was placed on anticoagulation therapy.

The stroke mechanism in this patient was thought to be a branch (the left SCA) atheromatous disease of the BA.

1-3. Hemodynamic (Low-Flow Type)

• Case 42

A 71-year-old right-handed man was referred from a local hospital with recurrent blindness of the left eye, which had developed 1 year ago. The symptoms occurred whenever he drank too much alcohol, took a sauna, or went hiking, and the duration was 2 hours on average. His medical history included hypertension, and hyperlipidemia. He was alert and his speech was normal. Motor power was all MRC grade V, and primary sensory modalities were normal. No bruit was heard on auscultation. Abnormal findings were not observed on laboratory tests. ECG and echocardiography were normal.

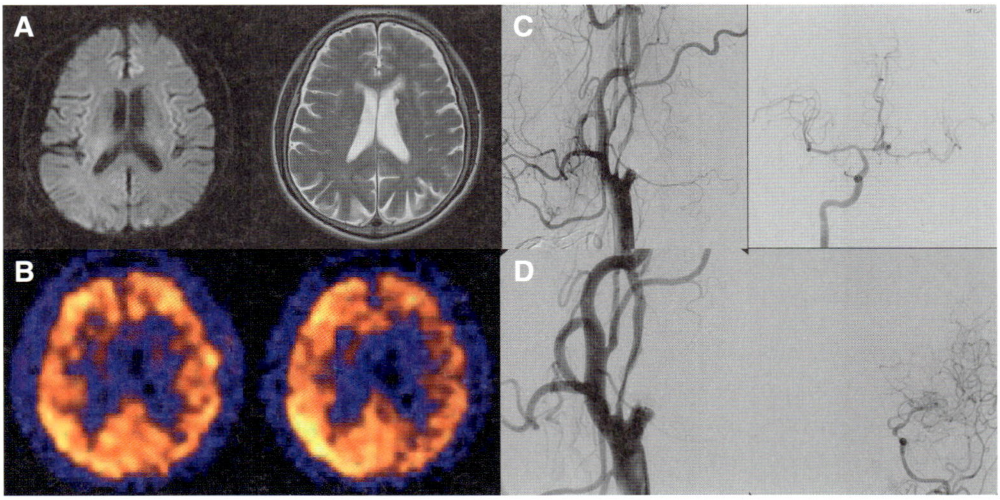

On brain DWI and T2WI, there were no acute and chronic infarctions (A). Brain SPECT (B) showed decreased vascular reserve in the left frontoparietal lobe. Conventional angiography (C) showed a near occlusion of the left ICA. The left MCA was partially supplied through the Acom. He underwent balloon angioplasty (D). All of his symptoms resolved after angioplasty.

The most common cause of transient monocular blindness is atherothromboembolism from the origin of the internal carotid artery (ICA), whereas atrial fibrillation is quite uncommon.[13] However, the prolonged reversible monocular loss of vision in this patient was likely to be a low flow phenomenon. Vision loss due to a near or complete occlusion of the ICA is characteristically associated with attacks being provoked by bright lights, altitudinal onset, and the occurrence of more than 10 attacks.[13] In this case, the ischemic stroke type was thought to be a low flow phenomenon because of the frequent attacks, onset specific situation (alcohol intake), and no acute lesions on DWI.

• Case 43

A 54-year-old woman visited our hospital for left-sided weakness and paresthesia while bathing on the day of admission. 8 days before admission, sudden blindness of right eye had occurred for 6 hours. He also felt a transient left-sided numbness and dysarthria 5 days before. He had dysarthria, but motor and sensory examinations were normal. Carotid bruit was inaudible. Holter monitoring and echocardiography did not reveal arrhythmia.

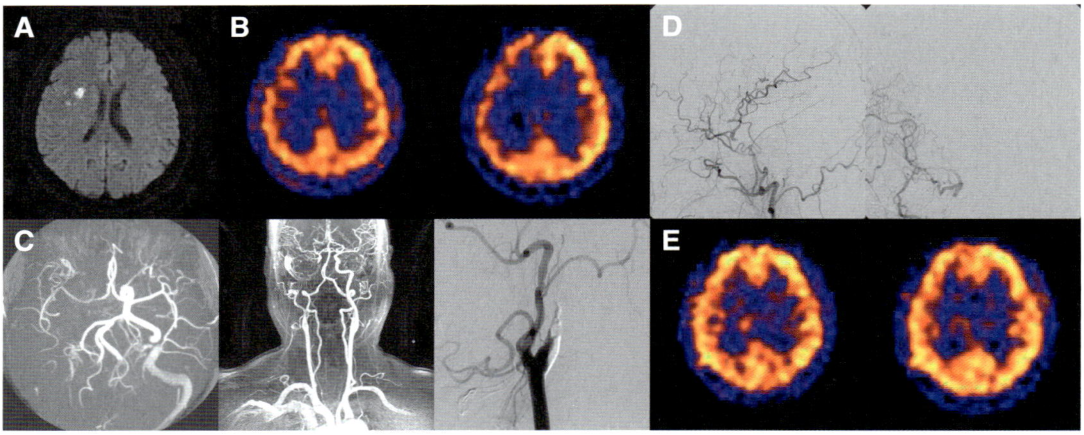

There were acute multifocal infarctions in the frontal lobes on DWI (A). However, brain SPECT (B) showed significantly decreased perfusion and vascular reserve in the right frontoparietal subcortical lesion. On brain MRA and conventional angiography (C), there was an occlusion of the right ICA. The right MCA was supplied through the Acom and posterior circulation. He underwent immediate STA-MCA bypass surgery (D). Follow-up brain SPECT at 6 months after bypass surgery showed much improved perfusion in the right hemisphere (E). His symptoms did not recur during a 12-month follow-up.

The stroke subtype was thought to be a low flow phenomenon considering the onset situation, relatively long duration of monocular blindness, and ICA occlusion with a profound decrease of perfusion. Early STA-MCA bypass may be beneficial in patients with acute strokes or strokes in progress. Furthermore, it appears safe when the infarction is small. The stroke rate after bypass surgery is reported to be 8% per year, which is favorable compared with an 18% rate reported for patients with internal carotid artery occlusion and impaired cerebrovascular reserve.[14]

• Case 44

A 77-year-old right-handed man came to our hospital due to left-sided weakness. He had a 15-year medical history of hypertension and diabetes mellitus and an acute myocardial infarction 3 years ago. However, he had not experienced any stroke symptoms until he suffered nausea and vomiting followed by a sudden left-sided weakness during breakfast on the day of admission. He also felt a left-sided numbness and dysarthria, but did not have headache, visual loss or mental change. He had a left facial palsy, limb weakness (MRC grade IV), and dysarthria. But, the examinations for sensation and deep tendon reflexes were normal. Mini-mental status examination was within normal limits. Carotid bruit was inaudible. Holter monitoring did not reveal arrhythmia, but echocardiography showed apicoanterior wall akinesia with aneurismal change.

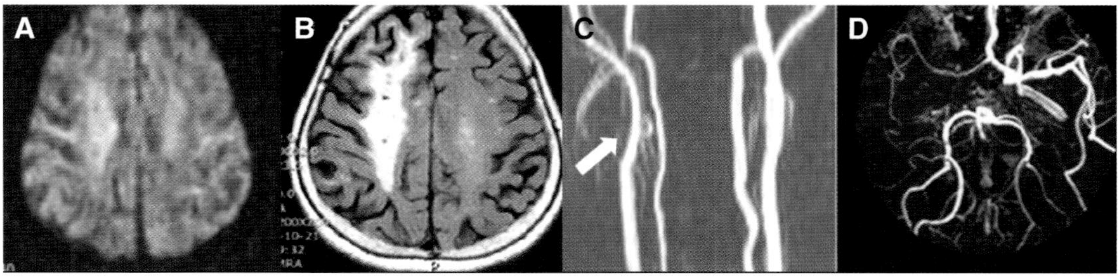

On brain MR-DWI (A), there was no acute infarction on DWI, but there was a diffuse frontoparietal subcortical lesion on FLAIR (B) corresponding to the ACA-MCA borderzone and internal borderzone. Brain MRA (C, D) showed occlusion of the right ICA (arrow). The right MCA was partially supplied via the Acom. The right PCA was brighter than the left PCA. Brain SPECT showed decreased vascular reserve in the right frontoparietal lobe. He had taken aspirin since his myocardial infarction, and the treatment was changed to intravenous heparinization. All of his symptoms disappeared 1 week later.

This ischemic stroke type was thought to be a low flow phenomenon because of the fuzzy incomplete infarct in the territory of the ICA borderzone, onset situation (eating), and patchy lesion on FLAIR imaging. The right ICA was likely to be occluded chronically. The right PCA signal was prominent due to increased cerebral blood flow from the leptomeningeal collateral circulation to the MCA territory.

• Case 45

A 71-year-old right handed man was admitted via a local hospital with a right hand weakness, aphasia and apraxia, which developed 2 months ago. His medical history included hypertension, diabetes mellitus, and hyperlipidemia. 5 years before, he had suffered from a left-sided weakness and left visual field defect. On neurologic examination, he had decreased fluency in speech, but intact repetition. He could obey one step commands, and showed dressing apraxia. Motor powers were all MRC grade V, and primary sensory modalities were normal. Dyscalculia and balint features were detected. On laboratory tests, abnormal findings were not observed. ECG and echocardiography were normal.

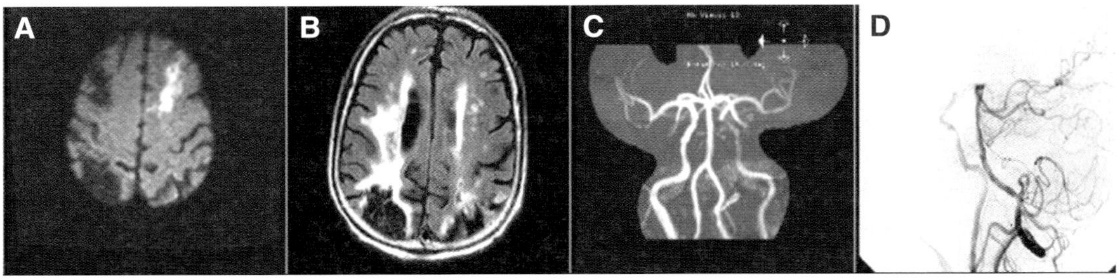

Brain MRI (A, B) showed an acute left ACA-MCA borderzone infarct and old infarcts of both MCA-PCA borderzone territories. Brain MRA (C) showed poor visualization of the left ICA flow and mild stenosis of the right distal ICA. On conventional angiography (D), his left CCA was occluded, and the left ICA flow was filled from the left VA via various collateral pathways. He was treated with aspirin and clopidogrel. His right hand weakness was much improved, but his apraxia did not change.

The acute left frontal infarction and old left MCA-PCA borderzone infarction can be explained by the low flow phenomenon, though the old right frontal and parietal infarctions are thought to be due to an unknown artery to artery embolism. Left subclavian-CCA anastomosis would be beneficial for enhancing blood flow of the left anterior circulation, but the feasibility is questionable.

• Case 46

A 65-year-old man presented with a transient right-sided weakness with a duration of less than 10 minutes. He experienced this symptom three times over 3 days within 2 hours after meals. 10 years before, he had been diagnosed with a right MCA infarction due to left-sided weakness. 3 months before, he had already been diagnosed with a left MCA infarction that caused a right-sided weakness. Severe atheroma in the aortic arch had been detected, and he had been treated with warfarin. He had hypertension and bladder cancer. He was an ex-smoker of 45 packyears. He was alert but his speech was dysarthric. Language function was normal, but tactile neglect was detected. The right limbs were slightly weak (MRC grade IV) and both hands were ataxic. No bruit was heard on the auscultation. The results of ECG and transthoracic echocardiography were normal. Transesophageal echocardiography and CT angiogram revealed a severe atheroma in aortic arch. PT INR was 1.84.

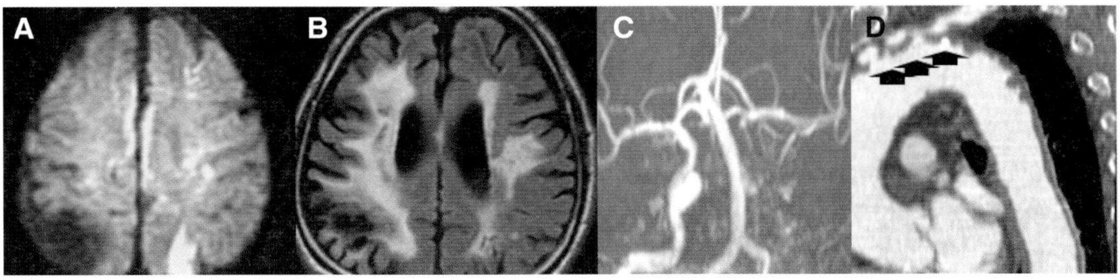

Brain MR-DWI (A) showed an acute left borderzone infarction. Old massive cerebromalacia in right MCA territory was noted on FLAIR imaging (B). Brain MRA (C) showed a left proximal ICA occlusion. CT angiography (D) revealed a severe atheroma in aortic arch (arrows). He was treated with heparin for a few days and the dose of warfarin was elevated to the target range of INR 2 to 3. There were no similar symptoms after meals in the ward. He was discharged.

Because of the occlusion of the left ICA, the left cerebral hemisphere was thought to be susceptible to hemodynamic change of the cerebral circulation. Recurrent symptoms only after meals suggest transient cerebral ischemia resulted from postprandial redistribution of blood flow.[15] The mechanism of stroke was low-flow. As for the old ischemic lesion in the right MCA territory, an artery to artery embolism from the aortic arch is also a possible mechanism.

• Case 47

A 53-year-old man visited our hospital for medical advice for his right-sided numbness. 5 years ago, he had experienced a sudden right-sided weakness for 2 hours, and heard from a neurologist when he was staying in the USA that his symptom was a TIA. He did not have any symptoms thereafter, but occasionally he felt right-sided numbness especially after cigarette smoking. During the last several months, he noted insidiously progressive dysarthria and more aggravated right-sided numbness. He was a current smoker of 30 packyears, but did not have hypertension, diabetes mellitus and hyperlipidemia. There was no family history of stroke. He had a stable BP and regular heart beat without murmur. There was no carotid or ophthalmic bruit on auscultation. However, his right arm dropped a few inches after being out-stretched for 10 seconds. He had mild dysarthria and moderately decreased sense for pain, temperature, and vibration on the right side. Transthoracic echocardiography and Holter monitoring did not reveal any cardiac sources of embolism.

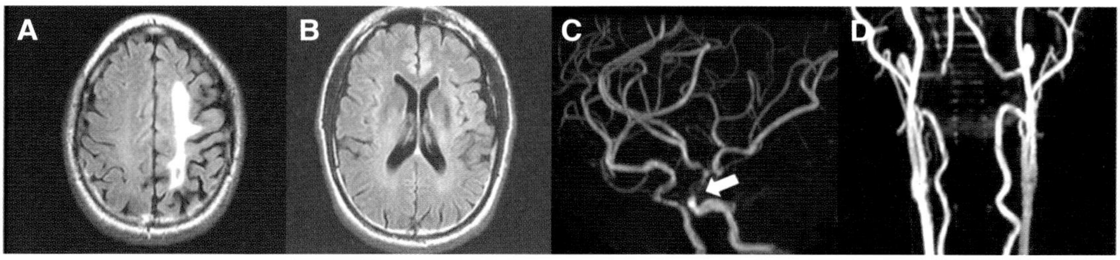

Brain MRI (A, B) showed chronic infarction in the left ACA-MCA borderzone and diffuse cerebral atrophy in the left hemisphere. Brain MRA (C, D) showed a decreased vascularity in the left MCA and ACA associated with a severe stenosis of the distal ICA (arrow). There was no stenosis in the proximal ICA. His symptoms of right side numbness and dysarthria had waxed and waned according to heavy smoking. He was prescribed antiplatelet agents, aspirin and clopidogrel. Angioplasty was recommended.

He is considered to have a low flow type infarction in borderzone area between the left MCA and ACA. His symptom fluctuation can be explained by a decreased cerebral blood flow due to vasoconstriction and hypoxia evoked by episodes of heavy smoking.

• Case 48

A 59-year-old woman had suffered from chronic hypertension and angina. She was also taking oral hypoglycemic agents due to diabetes mellitus for 4 years. 6 days before admission, she had experienced a right veering tendency at a sauna that lasted a few hours and then completely recovered. 2 days before, she had felt the same symptom while exercising. On neurological examination, she showed right-sided limb ataxia. There was a right veering tendency while walking. Transthoracic echocardiography and Holter monitoring did not reveal any cardiac sources of embolism.

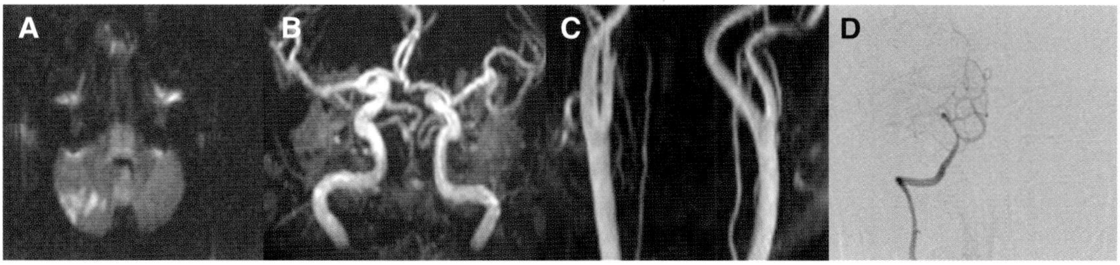

Brain MR-DWI (A) showed an acute right PICA infarction. Brain MRA (B, C) showed bilateral vertebrobasilar hypoplasia and that both PCAs were supplied by the anterior circulation. Conventional angiography (D) confirmed a severe stenosis in both distal VAs with indistinct continuation to the BA. She was medicated with a combination of clopidogrel and aspirin and discharged with slightly improved symptoms.

She had a right PICA territory stroke due to severe steno-occlusion of the VA. The ischemic stroke mechanism was thought to be a low flow type due to severe vertebrobasilar stenosis at the base of the right hypoplastic VA and the history of the precipitating clinical events.

• Case 49

A 48-year-old right handed man came to our hospital for a sudden right-sided weakness. He had a medical history of left thalamic intracerebral hemorrhage with intraventricular hemorrhage 5 years ago, and was diagnosed with hypertension, hyperlipidemia, and an occlusion of the left distal ICA at that time. He had been treated with triflusal and atorvastatin and had not suffered any sequelae. 1 day before admission, he realized a mild right limb weakness on awakening. On the next day, he could not speak well. There were no abnormal findings on the routine laboratory tests including hematocrit, fibrinogen, coagulation battery, etc. He showed a right central-type facial palsy, limb weakness (MRC grade IV), and motor-dominant aphasia. He had no cardiogenic embolic sources on the echocardiography.

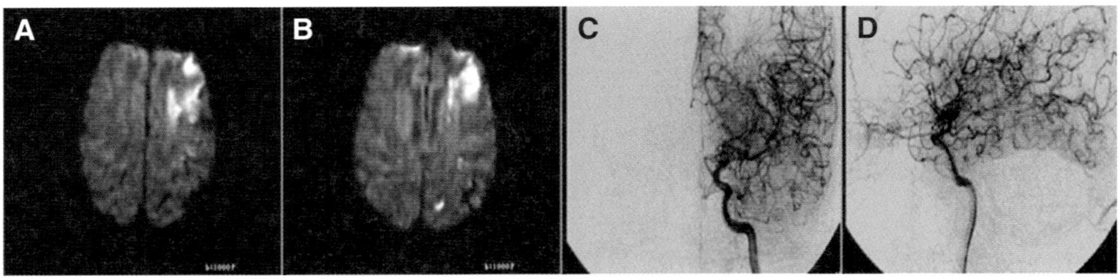

Brain MR-DWI (A, B) showed multiple acute infarctions in the left frontal and parietal lobes. Conventional angiography (C, D) showed complete occlusion of the left distal ICA with pericallosal and basal collaterals. Brain SPECT showed perfusion decrease with vascular reserve decrease in the left hemisphere. His symptoms were stationary with anticoagulation. Brain SPECT showed consistently decreased vascular reserve in the left MCA territory. He was referred to a neurosurgeon who performed STA-MCA bypass surgery 1 year later.

He had severe hemodynamic compromise to the left hemisphere. Although there was no definite clinical history of provoking low flow events, the most probable mechanism was thought to be a low flow stroke with or without small cortical embolic infarctions due to unilateral Moyamoya syndrome. The previous ICH with IVH was thought to have occurred due to the fragile Moyamoya vessels. STA-MCA bypass surgery should be carefully considered in these cases.

1-4. Combined Type

• Case 50

A 60-year-old man visited the emergency room because of a sudden left-sided weakness, which had developed 1 hour prior to his visit. He had no stroke risk factors, except diabetes mellitus. He was slightly drowsy. His speech was dysarthric. On examination, mild weakness involving the face and limbs on the left side (MRC grade IV) as well as hypesthesia on the same side were detected. The initial NIHSS was 8. ECG and transthoracic echocardiography revealed no abnormalities. HbA1c was 6.7%.

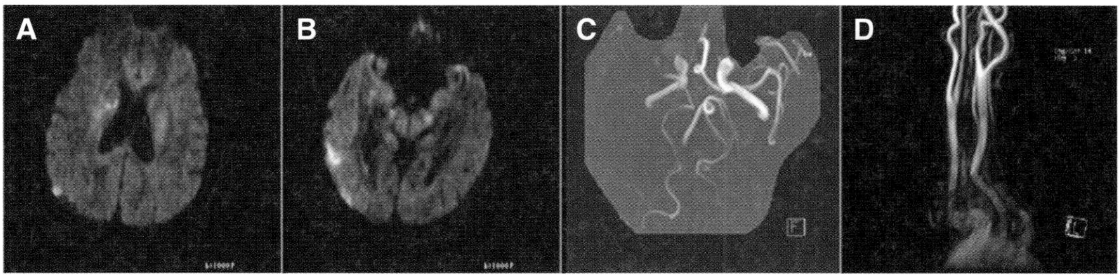

Brain MR-DWI (A, B) showed acute infarcts in the right temporal areas and basal ganglia. Brain MRA (C) showed non-visualization of the right MCA and right PCA supplied by the right ICA via the Pcom. Neck angiography (D) was normal. He was treated with intravenous thrombolysis, but his left hemiparesis progressed. In addition, sensory neglect and a visual field defect newly developed. The NIHSS increased from 8 to 12 within 1 day. Afterwards his symptoms were stationary, and he was discharged with antiplatelet agents.

The occlusion of the right MCA might result in acute infarctions of the perforator zone and artery to artery embolisms to the posterior temporal areas. The other areas were spared due to collateral flow. The stroke mechanism was thought to be an in situ thrombosis and an artery to artery embolization.

• Case 51

A 42-year-old woman presented with a headache and right-sided weakness that started one day. She had no history of hypertension, diabetes mellitus, and hyperlipidemia. Her mental status was alert. Cranial nerve examination showed a right homonymous hemianopsia. Her facial expression and sensation were normal. She showed mild dysarthria. The motor power of the right side was MRC grade IV in upper and lower extremities. Sensory examination revealed a right-sided hypesthesia in all modalities. Toe signs were both flexor. FBS and HbA1c were 131mg/dL and 5.4%. ECG, echocardiography and Holter monitoring showed no abnormal findings.

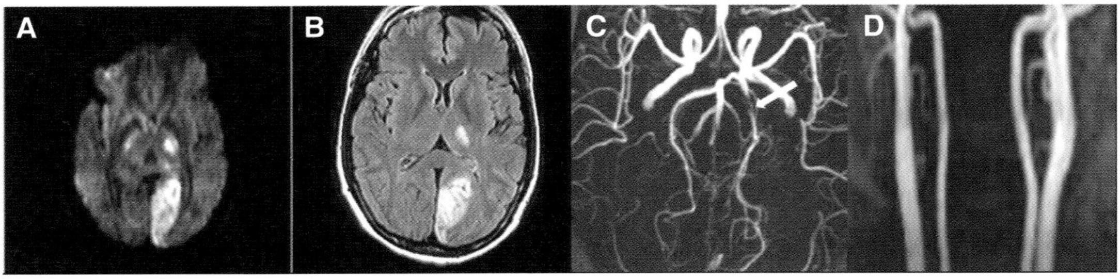

Brain MRI (A, B) showed an acute infarction in the left PCA territory. Brain MRA (C, D) showed a focal stenosis of the left PCA (arrow). The patient was initially treated with argatroban at a local hospital. 1 week later, he was treated with aspirin with clopidogrel.

There was no overt risk factor for stroke on history taking and examination. But there was a left PCA stenosis and left M2 stenosis on TCD and brain MRA. Therefore, the stroke mechanism might be an in situ thrombosis of the left PCA and a distal artery to artery embolism.

• Case 52

A 60-year-old man felt a sudden vertiginous sense and diplopia on waking. He had no weakness and sensory abnormalities. He didn't complain of headache, nausea, or vomiting. He had had a previous stroke left ACA infarction 1 year before, and been taking aspirin 300mg daily. Thereafter, he had sometimes complained of vertigo lasting for a few minutes along with perspiration. He had diabetes mellitus and hypertension. He was a current smoker of 40 packyears and a social drinker. His mental status was alert and intact. Cranial nerve examinations did not reveal any abnormal findings. He had a mild weakness of the right arm without sensory changes. Deep tendon reflexes of all four extremities were not increased. He showed a bilateral veering tendency on tandem gait. Echocardiography revealed no abnormal findings except sinus bradycardia. Fasting blood glucose was 138mg/dL, PP2 was 239mg/dL, and HbA1C was 7.2%. Low density lipoprotein cholesterol was 150mg/dL.

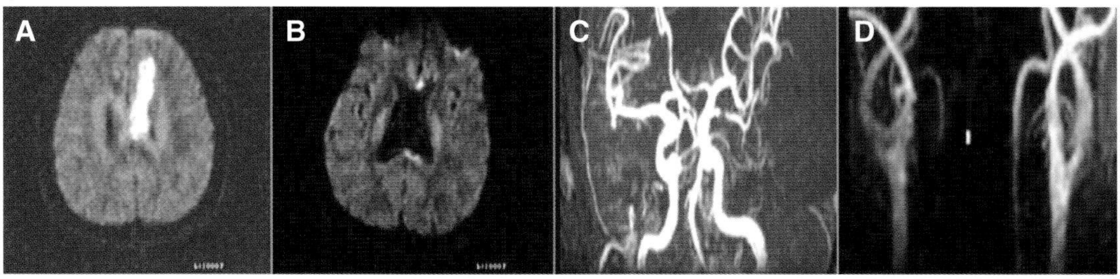

Brain MR-DWI (A, B) revealed recurrent ischemic events over 1 year. The first attack was in the left corpus callosum and the second attack was in the anterior and posterior corpus callosum. Brain MRA (C, D) showed total occlusion of the left A2 and a left P2 focal stenosis. Despite taking antiplatelet agents, a new stroke recurred, and thus we started him on short-term anticoagulation.

He had a history of hypertension, diabetes mellitus, a previous stroke and smoking. Images revealed a left corpus callosum infarction with a left ACA occlusion, but no proximal arterial stenosis. The mechanism may be an in situ thrombosis of the ACA in the first attack and an embolic infarction of the distal anterior cerebral artery in the second attack.

• Case 53

An 82-year-old right-handed man presented with a drowsy mentality and left-sided weakness, which was developed 3 hours before admission. He had atrial fibrillation and a 50-pack-year smoking history. His mental state was drowsy. He showed a gaze preponderance to the left. Motor power was MRC grade II on the left side. Sensory examination revealed a decreased withdrawal response on the left side. Deep tendon reflexes showed hyperreflexia on the left side. Echocardiography revealed left atrium enlargement without thrombi.

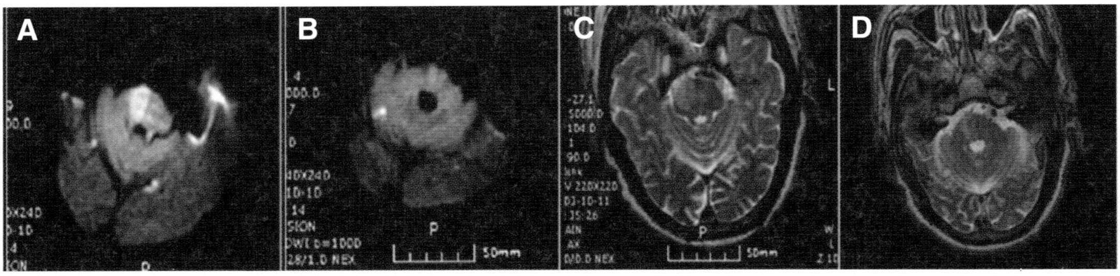

Brain MR-DWI (A, B) showed an acute infarction in the right pons, right SCA, and both PCA territories. T2WI (C, D) showed an irregular signal void of the vertebrobasilar system with intact blood flow. He showed bilateral weakness and his respiratory pattern was shallow. He was treated in the ICU for an extended period of time.

The patient did not present with a typical pontine lacune. The pontine lesion was large and located somewhat laterally. The pontine and right SCA infarction might be due to a basilar thrombosis. Bilateral PCA infarctions were due to artery to artery embolisms.

• Case 54

A 79-year-old man came to our hospital due to a sudden right-sided weakness. He had a 30-year history of diabetes mellitus. 2 hours before visiting the hospital, he felt a right-sided weakness during standing while urinating. Right-sided numbness and dysarthria also developed at that time. He was alert. Cranial nerve examinations showed no abnormal findings except a right central-type facial palsy and dysarthria. There was a right-sided limb weakness (MRC grade IV) and hypesthesia. Babinski sign was positive on the right. Transthoracic echocardiography and Holter monitoring did not reveal any cardiac sources of embolism.

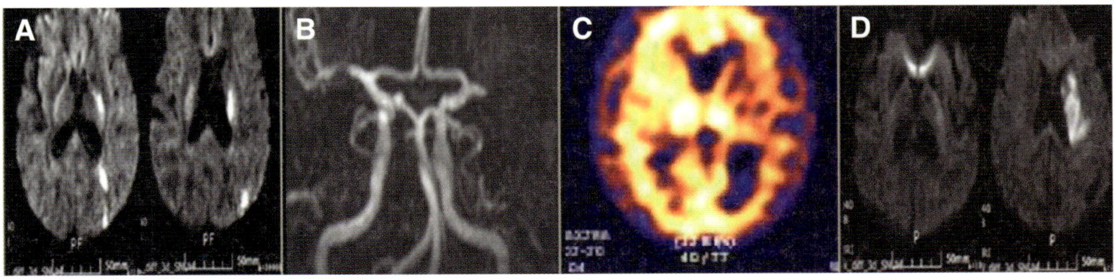

Brain MR-DWI (A) showed multiple small acute ischemic infarctions in the left paraventricular area, left posterior frontal cortex, and whiter matter of the left frontal lobe and left parietooccipital area, mainly in the watershed area. Brain MRA (B) showed complete occlusion or severe stenosis of the left MCA stem, and mild narrowing of the right MCA at M1 segment. Brain SPECT (C) showed a perfusion defect and decreased reserve in the left fronto-temporo-parietal cortex. Initially he was treated with aspirin. At the eighth hospital day, involuntary movement of the right limb developed and diffusion MR showed extension of the infarction into the left periventricular white matter (D). So, the treatment was changed to a aspirin-clopidogrel combination.

The stroke mechanism was firstly an artery to artery embolization from the left MCA with subsequent extension of the in situ thrombosis in the left MCA stem.

• Case 55

A 64-year-old man presented with dysphagia and dizziness, which suddenly developed 7 days ago. He had suffered from hypertension for 5 years. He was a current smoker of 40 pack-years. He was alert and oriented. Cranial nerve examinations showed ptosis and miosis of the right eye and facial hypesthesia on the right. Dysphagia and dysarthria were also present. Motor power was intact but hypesthesia of the left hemibody was detected. He also had limb ataxia on the right. ECG and echocardiography showed no abnormalities.

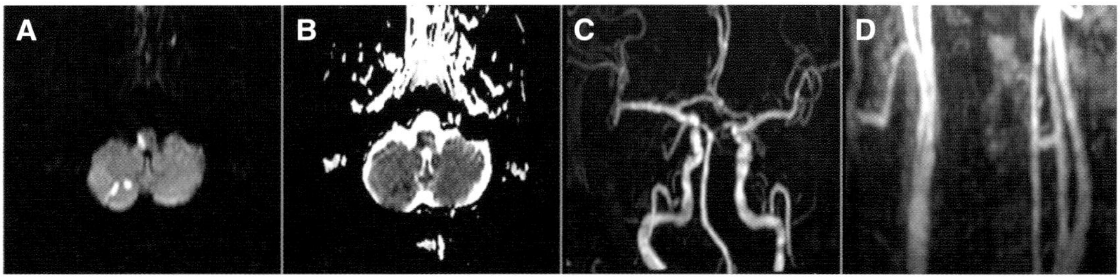

Brain DWI and ADC map (A, B) showed acute multifocal infarctions in the right inferior cerebellum and right lateral medulla. Brain MRA (C, D) showed non-visualization of the right VA. He was treated with anticoagulation. Soon after the stroke, his admission was complicated by aspiration pneumonia. Swallowing difficulty persisted at the time of discharge, while other symptoms improved.

The mechanism of stroke was thought to be an in situ thrombosis of the VA with an artery to artery embolization to the distal PICA. About 13% of lateral medullary infarcts are associated with PICA territory cerebellar infarcts.[11] Dysphagia appears to be more severe in rostral lesions of the lateral medulla and tend to persist longer than other symptoms probably due to impaired sensory input from the oropharynx as well as pharyngeal paralysis resulting from involvement of the nucleus ambiguus.[16]

• Case 56

A 43-year-old man was hospitalized for recurrent left-sided weakness. His symptoms lasted about 5 minutes and had developed six times during the past 2 months. His left-sided weakness persisted for 3 days before admission. He had no history of hypertension, diabetes mellitus, dyslipidemia, and smoking. The motor powers of the left limbs were both grade III. Deep tendon reflexes of the left side were increased. Echocardiography and Holter monitoring showed normal findings. Rheumatoid factor and anti-La antibody were positive, but there was no other evidence of Sjogren syndrome.

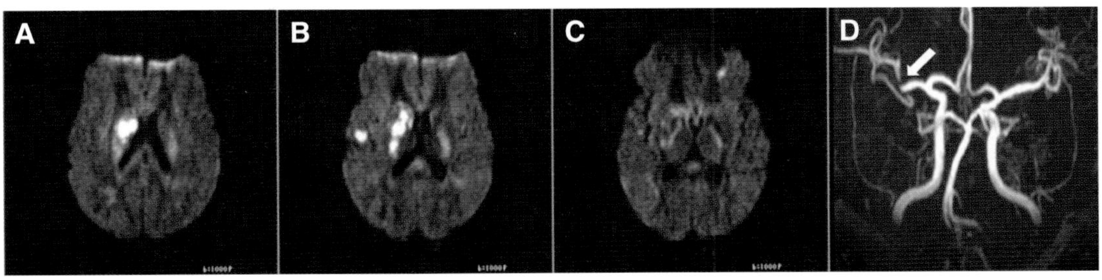

Brain MR-DWI (A-C) showed acute infarcts in the right periventricular white matter, right basal ganglia and right temporal lobe. Brain MRA (D) revealed a right M2 stenosis (arrow). We started the patient on anticoagulation and performed vasculitis labs, but we did not find any factors for young age stroke.

The stroke mechanisms were embolic TIAs initially and then embolic and/or in situ thrombotic stroke. The etiology is possibly related to vasculitis, but the exact cause is still undetermined.

• Case 57

A 44-year-old man developed a right-sided weakness, dysarthria, and abnormal behavior at 4 days before admission. He had been diagnosed as hypertension, but had not taken antihypertensive medication. He was a 40-pack-year smoker. At first, he visited a local hospital and was given Urokinase intravenously. His mental status was confused. The disorientation for time and place was observed. The right-sided hypesthesia was detected. And the motor power of the right side was MRC grade IV. Echocardiography showed no abnormal findings.

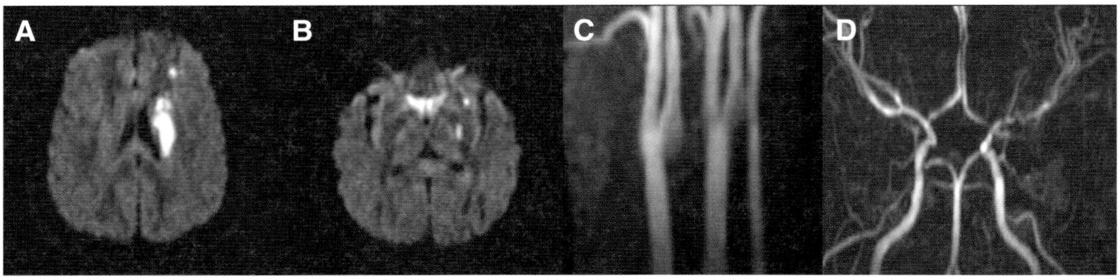

Brain MR-DWI (A, B) showed acute infarcts in the left MCA territory involving basal ganglia and subcortical WM. Brain MRA (C, D) showed a severe focal stenosis of the left M1 and a decreased vascularity of the left MCA. We started antiplatelet agent, and his symptoms were slowly improved.

The stroke mechanism of this patient was in situ thrombosis with an artery to artery embolism from the proximal MCA.

• Case 58

A 67-year-old, right-handed man presented with a sudden onset of left-sided weakness and dysarthria which was developed 2 hours prior to visit. He had a hypertension with regular medication for 8 months and was a current smoker with 40 packyears. He was alert and neglect was not revealed. Gaze preponderance to the right side and weakness involving limbs and face on the left side were detected. Carotid bruit on the left side was heard on auscultation. Transthoracic echocardiography and transesophageal echocardiography showed no source of embolism.

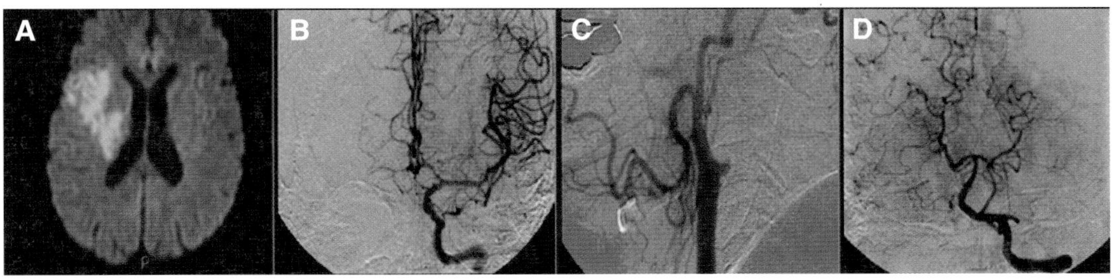

Brain MR-DWI (A) showed an acute infarction in the right MCA superior division. Conventional angiography (B-D) showed a collateral flow from the left ICA via Acom and from PCA via Pcom to right hemisphere and an occlusion of the right proximal ICA. Intraarterial thrombolysis was tried but failed. He was treated with an antiplatelet agent. Neurologic status was stationary.

The mechanism of stroke was thought to be an artery to artery embolism from the distal stump of the occluded right ICA. Areas with more flow from collateral circulation might be saved from the ischemic injury.

• Case 59

A 68-year-old man was admitted to emergency room because of a dysarthria and left-sided weakness on awakening. He had a history of diabetes mellitus and hypertension. Neurologic examination showed a gaze preponderance to the right and left facial palsy of the central type. Strength of the left arm was MRC grade I and that of the left leg was grade III. Tactile extinction was observed on his left side. Hyperreflexia and Babinski sign was observed in the left side. Transesophageal echocardiography showed atheromatous plaques on the descending thoracic aorta.

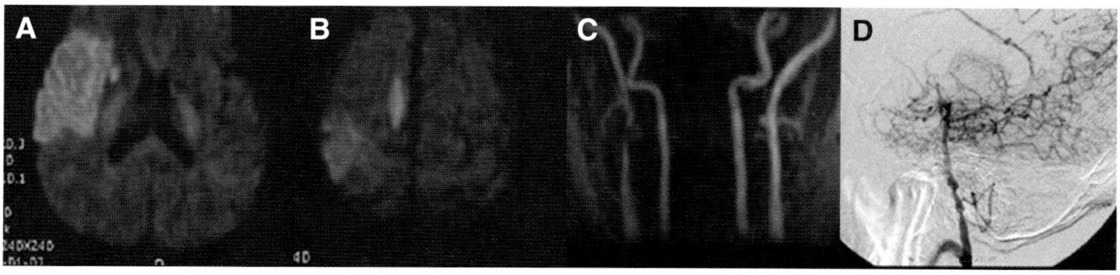

Brain MR-DWI (A, B) showed right parieto-temporal acute infarction and right ACA infarction. Brain MRA (C, D) revealed total occlusion of both ICAs and intracranial posterior circulation only. Although he had a severe carotid stenosis bilaterally, leptomeningeal collateral supplies from posterior circulation were relatively intact. He was discharged with a sequallae of left hemiparesis.

This patient had totally occluded ICAs, and was hemodynamically unstable. However, given the infarctions were distributed in the right ACA and MCA territory, an artery to artery embolism from right ICA may be responsible for the mechanism of stroke. Embolus may fall into the MCA or ACA just before the definite occlusion of the "nearly occluded carotid artery" or embolizations can be developed to the distal arteries by the rupture of the right proximal ICA atheroma with subsequent occlusion of the vessel.

• Case 60

A 76-year-old man visited our emergency room for a sudden weakness of the left limbs. 2 hours before admission, he had noticed left-sided weakness and dysarthria at awaking. He did not have any remarkable past medical history. He was a social drinker, and ex-smoker of 35 packyears. His emergency routine laboratory tests, however, revealed elevated fasting glucose and HbA1c. He showed stable vital sign and normal sinus rhythm. In the motor power examination, he could not move his left arm, but could slightly lift his left leg. He showed a left central-type facial palsy, and gaze preponderance to the right side. However, he could feel intact sense to pain stimuli. Carotid bruit was not audible on both sides, and transthoracic echocardiography and Holter monitoring showed normal findings.

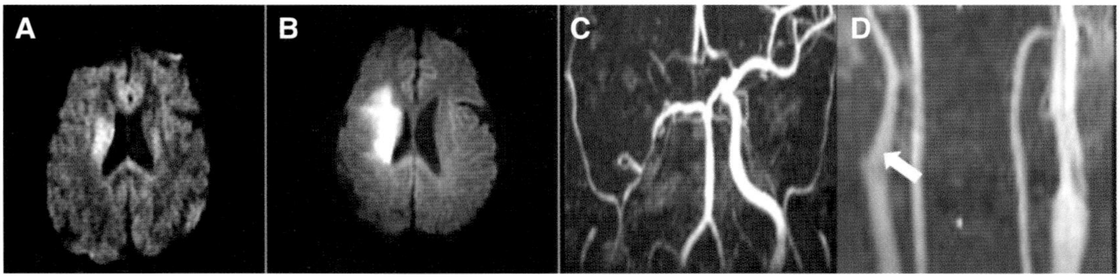

Initial brain MR-DWI (A) showed acute infarctions in the right insula, basal ganglia, and corona radiata. Next day, he could not move the left leg at all, and showed hemi-neglect on the right. Follow-up image (B) showed an extension of T2 lesion in the periventricular area. Brain MRA (C, D) showed nonvisualization of right ICA from the CCA bifurcation, and right ACA was supplied by Acom with another occlusion of the right proximal M1. He was treated with dual antiplatelet agents.

His brain MRA indicated that the right proximal ICA had been occluded, and the right ICA territory was supplied by the opposite ACA through Acom. We think that he had another tandem stenotic lesion on the right M1, resulting in acute right striatocapsular infarction. As the stenosis of the right MCA progressed, the right MCA internal watershed zone was likely to be injured by decreased collateral perfusion. The blurred T2 high signal area of centrum semiovale must be the internal borderzone of the right MCA between the lenticulostriate arteries and pial arteries.

• Case 61

A 76-year-old, right-handed man presented with a sudden onset of inappropriate speaking, which was developed 4 days prior to visit. He had no risk factors for stroke. He had a bladder cancer. He was alert but showed word-finding difficulty, acalculia and right-left disorientation. Mild weakness involving the right face and ipsilateral arm was detected. ECG and transthoracic echocardiography showed no abnormal findings.

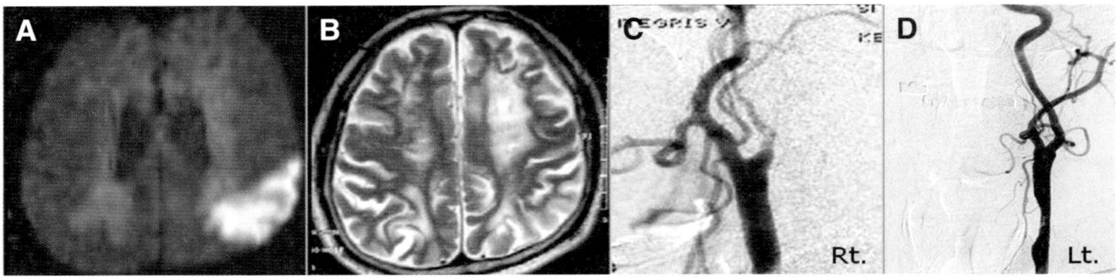

Brain MR-DWI (A) showed an acute infarction in the left inferior parietal lobe. T2WI (B) showed chronic confluent lesions in both PVWM. Conventional angiography showed a severe stenosis of the right proximal ICA (C) and the left midcervical CCA (D), and an ulcerated plague on the left carotid bulb (D). He was treated with anticoagulant and antiplatelet agent. Neurologic symptoms were improved and only acalculia was left when he was discharged.

The mechanism of stroke was thought to be an artery to artery embolism from the left proximal ICA or stenotic CCA. Old lesions involving bilateral internal borderzone and right parieto-occipital lobe might result from chronic low flow state and partly from small artery to artery embolisms.

2. Cardioembolism

• Case 62

A 70-year-old woman, who had a 10-year history of hypertension presented with a dysarthria and a left-sided weakness. She had had mitral valve regurgitation and had been operated for tissue valve replacement 6 years before. She had taken warfarin for 6 months after surgery, and changed it into aspirin. 1 day before admission, she had showed sudden dysarthria, left-sided weakness, and visuospatial dysfunction. She was alert, but can neither do simple calculation nor find out her house. However, her symptoms were much improved at emergency room. In mini-mental score examination, total score was 25, as minus in calculation (-3), recall (-1), and interlocking pentagon (-1) each. Neurologic examination confirmed the presence of mild left-sided facial palsy and dysarthria. Motor power in left limb was MRC grade IV. The patient had spontaneous echogenic contrast in the left atrium in transesophageal echocardiography.

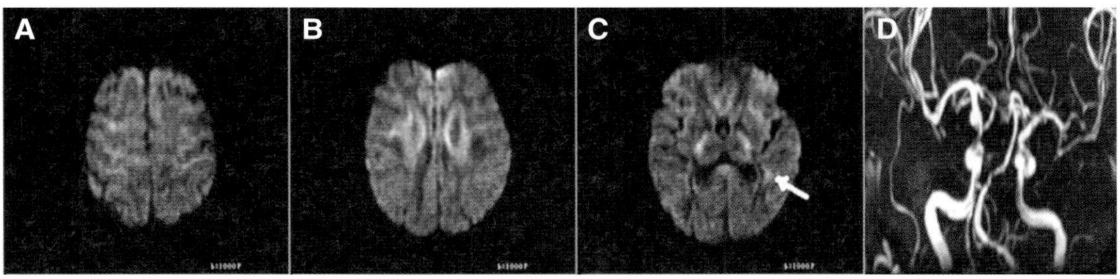

Brain MR-DWI (A-C) showed the right frontal cortical, left temporal subcortical, and right basal ganglia lesions. Brain MRA (D) showed focal stenoses in BA, right PCA, left MCA, and luminal narrowing in both distal ICAs. She was treated with heparin in suspect of cardioembolism, and afterwards, most of her symptoms were improved. Mini-mental status examination at discharge was 28.

She had mainly the right hemispheric symptoms. However, dyscalculia was left hemispheric symptom. Although she had a medium risk of cardioembolism (tissue valve replacement), the mechanism of stroke was presumed to be a cardioembolism because of bilateral DWI lesions and symptoms.

• Case 63

A 64-year-old woman presented with a left-sided weakness 1 hour ago. Medical history included hypertension, diabetes mellitus, mitral valve replacement 8 years ago, and recurrent left MCA infarction, 5 years and 2 years ago. She was also diagnosed to have Takayasu's arteritis. The mental status was deep drowsy. The cranial nerve examination showed right gaze preponderance and left central-type facial palsy. The motor power was MRC grade II on the left side, and MRC grade IV on the right lower extremity due to sequelae from the prior strokes. The sensory examination showed hypesthesia on left side. The deep tendon reflex was hyperreflexive on left side. Transthoracic echocardiography and transesophageal echocardiography showed dilated left atrium.

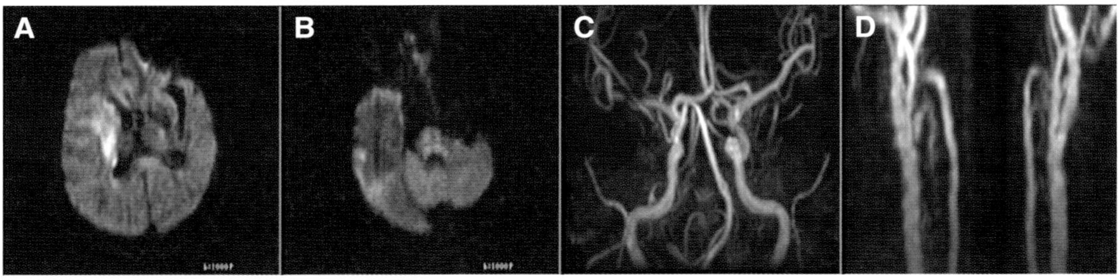

Brain MR-DWI (A, B) showed multiple high signal intensities in the right striatocapsular territory and small cortical lesions in right temporal area. Brain MRA (C, D) showed a focal stenosis of the right MCA. She was treated with anticoagulation due to mitral valve replacement and recurrent stroke episodes. The symptoms slowly improved.

Cardioembolic stroke was suggested in this patient. Takayasu's arteritis was not thought to be associated with the ischemic strokes.

• Case 64

A 73-year-old woman presented with a left limb weakness. She had a history of mitral stenosis with atrial fibrillation, which made her operated for valvuloplasty 12 years ago. She had no vascular risk factors such as hypertension, diabetes mellitus, hyperlipidemia or smoking. 1 day prior to admission, she had experienced a sudden weakness in the middle of drinking. It persisted until next day, and was accompanied by mild dysarthria. Neurologic examination revealed a ptosis in the right eye and a central-type facial palsy in the left side. Motor power was MRC grade IV in the left upper and lower extremities, but the sensory loss was not observed. Routine laboratory findings were entirely normal, but ECG showed atrial fibrillation.

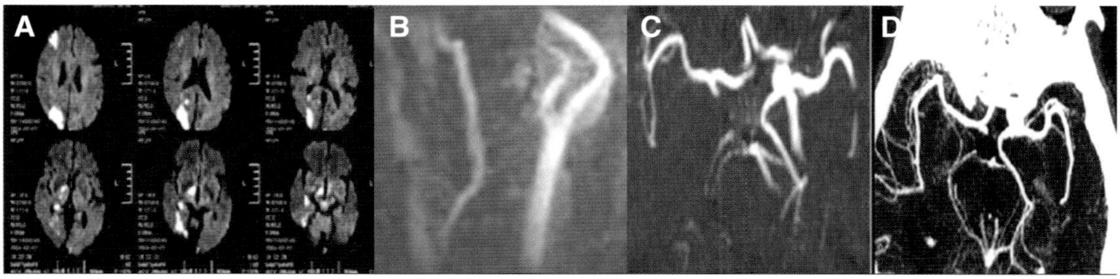

Brain MR-DWI (A) showed multiple infarctions in the frontal lobe, occipital lobe, thalamus and midbrain in the right hemisphere. There was a poor signal of the right CCA with ICA occlusion in the extracranial MRA (B). Intracranial MRA (C) did not visualize the right distal ICA and Pcom with a stenosis in the right proximal PCA. Pcom which was initially occluded by embolus from CCA was recanalized in the follow-up CT angiography (D). The motor weakness rapidly improved to MRC grade V until the follow-up CT angiography revealed faint right Pcom 2 days after initial MRA. He was managed with anticoagulation, and discharged in state of mild dysarthria and facial palsy.

The main flow of the right PCA seems to be originally supplied not by hypoplastic PCA, but Pcom, which was initially occluded by embolus from the fibrillating heart was recanalized in the follow-up CT angiography. The territory of thalamic infraction corresponded to thalamoperforating artery and posterior choroidal artery territory.

• Case 65

A 75-year-old woman was said to have atrial fibrillation with mitral stenosis. After percutaneous mitral valvuloplasty 5 years before, she had been medicated with aspirin. 6 days before admission, she had a sudden onset occipital headache and vertigo. On neurologic examination, she showed a left-sided dysmetria and dysdiadochokinesia. Echocardiography revealed moderate mitral stenosis and dilated left atrium with appendage sludge and suspected thrombi in left atrium apex.

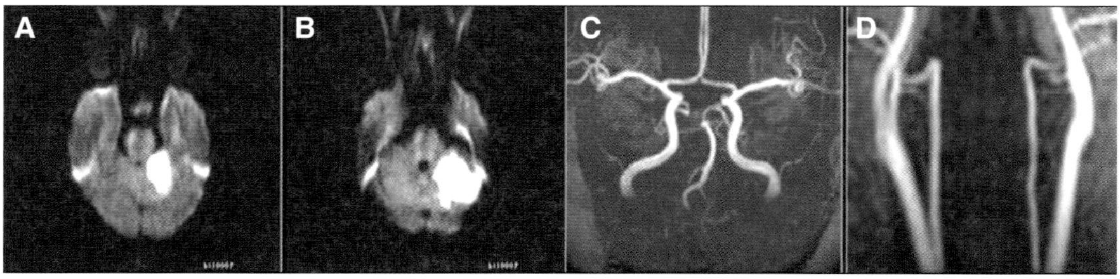

Brain MR-DWI (A, B) showed an acute infarct in the left SCA territory. Brain MRA (C, D) showed normal cerebral arteries. We treated him with anticoagulant, and his symptoms improved much.

He had a high-risk cardioembolic source. The mechanism of stroke must be a cardioembolism to the left SCA.

• Case 66

A 63-year-old man presented with a left-sided weakness, which is dominant in lower extremity 1 day ago. Medical history included hypertension for 20 years, diabetes mellitus for 2 years, hyperlipidemia and atrial fibrillation. He was a current smoker of 40 packyears. He had been treated with warfarin. For dental operation, he had discontinued warfarin for 5 days, and then, the neurologic symptoms developed. The cranial nerve examination showed no abnormal findings. The weakness on the left side was MRC grade III on upper extremity and MRC grade I on lower extremity. Sensory examination was normal, and deep tendon reflex was hyper-reflectic on the left. The echocardiographic examination showed spontaneous echogenic contrast and appendage sludge in left atrium.

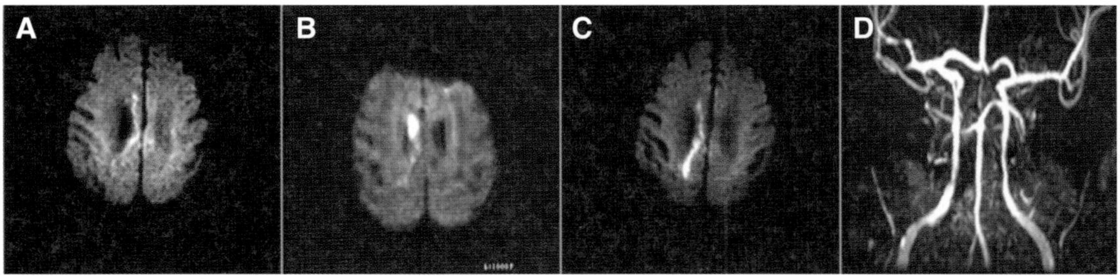

Brain MR-DWI (A, B) showed acute lesions in the right ACA territory. Anticoagulation was restarted. But a few weeks later, he suffered more progressive weakness on the left lower extremities with another high signal intensity of right corpus callosum in DWI (C). Brain MRA (D) showed right M2 multifocal stenosis and both distal ICA luminal irregularity.

The stroke mechanism was thought to be a cardioembolism, after discontinuation of warfarin for dental preparation, which did not respond well to re-starting of anticoagulation.

• Case 67

A 75-year-old man presented with a transient left-sided weakness. During walking around the park, he suddenly felt a left leg weakness and dysarthria. Weakness persisted for more than 30 minutes, and then recovered. He had had atrial fibrillation without management and was a current smoker of 40 packyears. At the time of admission, neurologic examination showed no abnormality. ECG showed atrial fibrillation. Spontaneous echogenic contrast and sludge were detected in the left atrium on the transesophageal echocardiography.

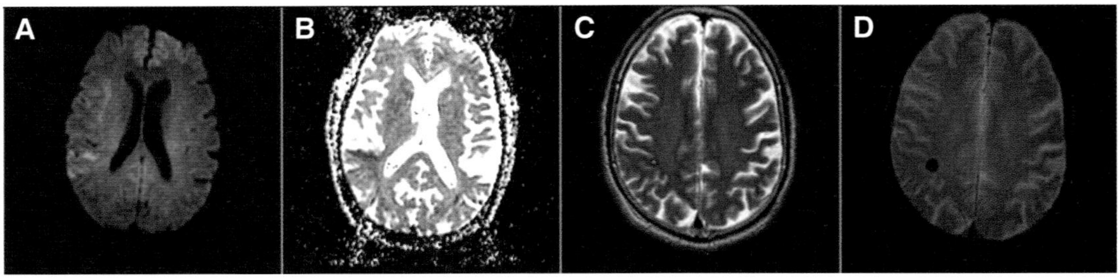

Brain MR-DWI and ACD map (A, B) revealed acute focal cortical infarction in the left MCA territory. T2W-MRI (C) and GRE image (D) identified the hemorrhagic spot around the lesion. We don't know whether the microbleed occurred with this clinical event or pre-existed, but we do know that some microbleeds can be developed with new stroke and disappear afterward. Brain MRA showed no significant abnormality. He was treated with anticoagulant. There was no further attack after anticoagulation.

The stroke mechanism was presumed to be a cardioembolism. The DWI abnormalities in TIA patients tend to be associated with symptoms lasted more than 1 hour.

• Case 68

A 55-year-old woman visited our hospital for a left-sided weakness developed 2 hours ago. Medical history included atrial fibrillation and hypertension. In the past medical history, she had undergone aneurysmal clipping surgery in the right Pcom 11 years ago. The mental status was drowsy. She showed right gaze preponderance, left central-type facial palsy, left side hemineglect, anosognosia and autotopagnosia. Motor power of the left side was MRC grade II. Echocardiography revealed left atrium enlargement without thrombi.

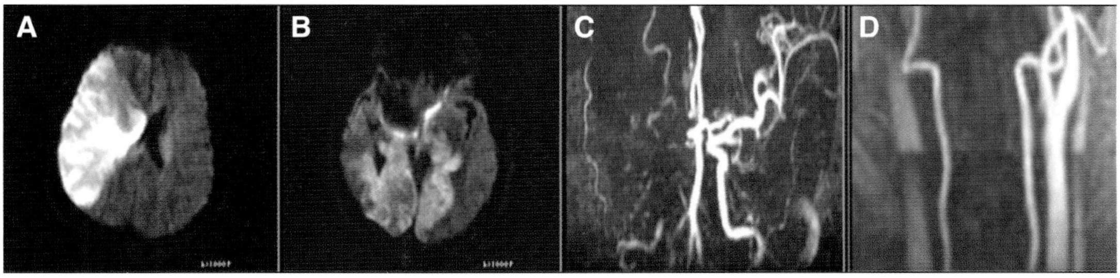

Brain MR-DWI (A) showed total infarction of the right MCA territory. Anticoagulation was started. But 1 month later, recurrent stroke developed with bilateral PCA and PICA territory (B). Rt ICA was not visualized on brain MRA (C, D), possibly due to flow stagnation of the right distal ICA embolic occlusion. After the recurred stroke, she became vegetative.

Recurrent large cardioembolism was the main stroke mechanism in this patient.

• Case 69

A 72-year-old woman presented with a sudden changed mentality. Other family members noticed that she was out of consciousness and her respiration was abnormal. She was transferred to our emergency room from other hospital in an intubated state. At emergency room, decerebrated tonic postures of four extremities were frequently seen. She had no history of diabetes mellitus or hypertension. She was semi-comatose. Both pupils were not reactive to light and the left third nerve palsy was detected. Brainstem reflexes except gag reflex were impaired. Babinski sign was positive bilaterally. Atrial fibrillation was detected on ECG. Left atrium was dilated on transthoracic echocardiography, and transesophageal echocardiography could not be done.

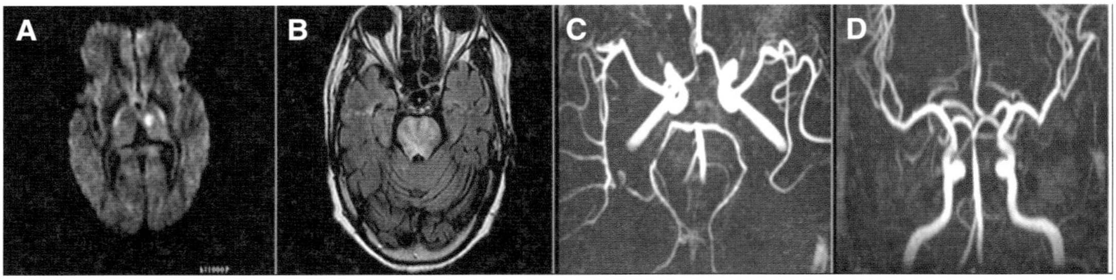

Brain MR-DWI (A, B) showed acute multifocal infarct in pons, left thalamus, and midbrain. Brain MRA (C, D) showed no significant stenosis except for the right distal PCA stenosis. The radiologic findings indicate massive basilar embolization with relatively rapid recanalization. She was taken care of in ICU with mechanical ventilator and anticoagulation. Weaning of ventilator was done but her mentality showed no improvement.

She had a definite high risk source of cardioembolism and no other stroke risk factor. The stroke mechanism was a cardioembolism by atrial fibrillation. The cardioembolism is frequently complicated by hemorrhagic conversion, which can make worse prognosis than without.

• Case 70

A 76-year-old man developed a right-sided weakness and loss of consciousness. After 5 minutes, he recovered alertness but showed decreased verbal output and dysarthria. Past medical history revealed no abnormalities. At admission, atrial fibrillation was found on ECG and Holter monitoring. Neurological examination showed a mild right-sided weakness and dysarthria. No further abnormal finding was found in his cardiac evaluations

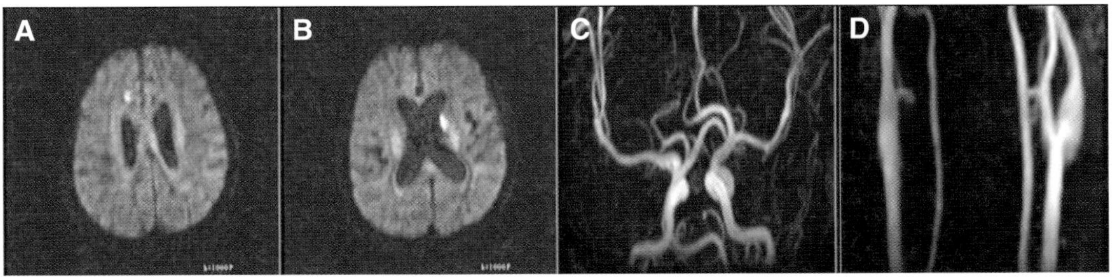

Brain MR-DWI (A, B) showed small acute infarcts in the left basal ganglia and in the right frontal lobe. Brain MRA (C, D) showed no significant stenosis. His neurological symptoms were fully recovered.

The stroke mechanism of this patient was a cardioembolism by lone atrial fibrillation.

• Case 71

A 70-year-old man presented with dizziness on the day of visit. The dysarthria and right falling tendency was accompanied. Medical history included atrial fibrillation and hypertension on regular medication for 10 years. Diabetes mellitus and hyperlipidemia were not present. The mental status was alert. The cranial nerve examination showed a head tilting to the left and downbeating nystagmus. The facial sensory and expression were normal. There was dysarthria. The motor power was all MRC grade V. The sensory and deep tendon reflex examinations were all within normal limits. The cerebellar function test showed right dysmetria and dysdiadochokinesia. The gait showed right falling tendency. The carotid/ophthalmic bruits were inaudible. The FBS/HbA1c and lipid panel were within normal range. Transthoracic echocardiography and transesophageal echocardiography showed dilated left atrium.

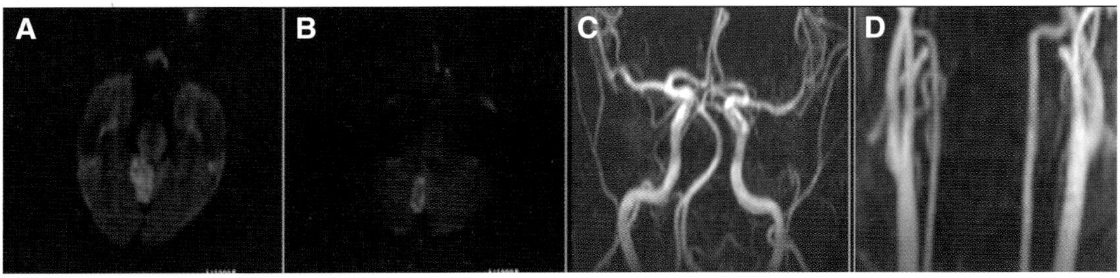

Brain MR-DWI (A, B) showed an acute infarction in right SCA territory. Brain MRA (C, D) showed no significant stenoocclusive lesion. Anticoagulation was started, and then the symptoms slowly improved.

The cranial nerve examination showed a head tilting to the left, which was possibly due to midbrain tectal involvement. The cause of infarction in the right SCA territory in this patient was a cardioembolism, which is the main cause of SCA infarction.

• Case 72

A 73-year-old man visited emergency room because of the left facial palsy and dysarthria. He had a medical history of hypertension, diabetes mellitus and atrial fibrillation. 8 hours before visiting emergency room, he felt left facial palsy with dysarthria during drinking water. He was alert. Neurologic examination revealed the left central type facial palsy and dysarthria. Motor power and sensory functions were intact in four extremities.

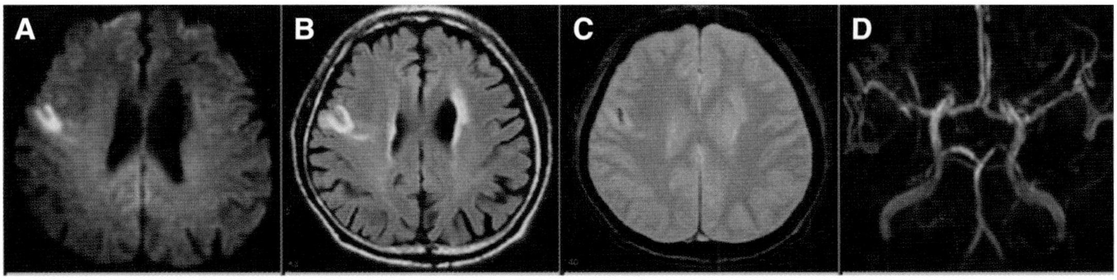

MRI (A, B) showed an acute small infarction in the right precentral gyrus. This lesion had minor hemorrhagic component evidenced by GRE image (C). Brain MRA (D) showed diffuse irregular vascular changes in both proximal MCA and left distal ICA at the cavernous segment. He was treated with heparin in suspect of cardioembolism, and afterward, his neurologic symptoms were improved.

The stroke mechanism was an embolic infarction of cardiac or arterial origin. One of the characteristic MR findings of the embolic infarct with early recanalization is cortical infarct along the neocortical mantle which is one of the most sensitive areas to ischemic insult. Hemorrhagic conversion is also a frequent finding of cardioembolism.

• Case 73

A 63-year-old man came to emergency room for a sudden left-sided weakness. He had had two stroke events 4 years before and last year each, which manifested also as sudden left-sided weakness. He had recovered with mild limping gait until recently with taking aspirin. He was found in drowsy and left hemiplegic state 3 hours prior to visiting E/R. He had a history of long-standing hypertension, 40-pack-year smoking and heavy drinking. He was in deep drowsy state, and had facial palsy, hemiplegia (MRC grade I), hypesthesia, and hemianopsia in the left side. Gaze preponderance to the right side was noted, but cortical symptoms were not able to check because of drowsy mental state. Carotid bruit was inaudible, but ECG revealed atrial fibrillation which had not been known.

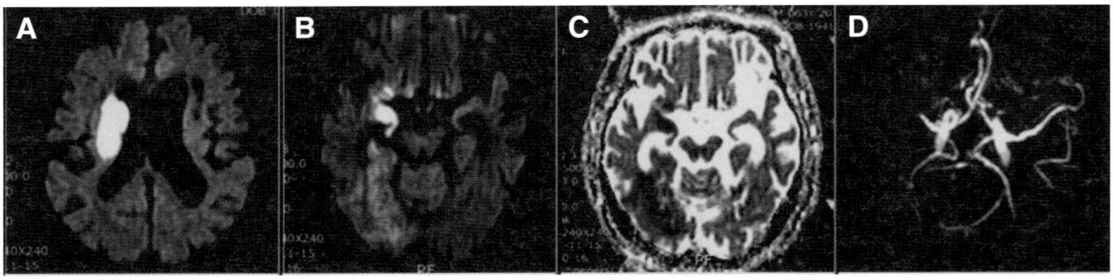

Brain MR-DWI (A-C) showed acute infarctions involving the right basal ganglia, medial temporal uncus, and occipital lobe. Brain MRA (D) revealed a right MCA occlusion, BA stenosis, both A2 stenosis, and bilateral fetal circulation. Warfarin was added to the antiplatelet medication.

There was a possibility of MCA disease in the right side, which could be inferred by two stroke episodes of left-sided weakness. However, the left hemianopsia with increased signal in the right occipital lobe, and medial temporal lesion which were corresponded to the left PCA and anterior choroidal artery territories, strongly suggested embolism transiently lodged in the distal right ICA migrating to the right MCA, PCA via Pcom, and possibly to anterior choroidal artery, too. He had a definite potential cardiogenic embolic source of atrial fibrillation.

• Case 74

A 73-year-old woman visited our hospital complaining of a sudden right-sided weakness and language disturbance. Mild mental change was associated, but headache and nausea were not. She had hypertension, diabetes mellitus and atrial fibrillation history with regular follow-up and medication through the clinic. On visiting hospital, BP was 140/90mmHg. On mental examination, she was mild drowsy and global aphasia was noted. Cranial nerve examination showed the right central-type facial palsy and dysphagia. And there was a right-sided weakness of MRC grade I and hypesthesia. Deep tendon reflex was increased in the right. ECG showed atrial fibrillation, but other serum laboratory tests were all normal range. Transthoracic echocardiography is normal, but transesophageal echocardiography revealed atheromatous plaque in descending aorta.

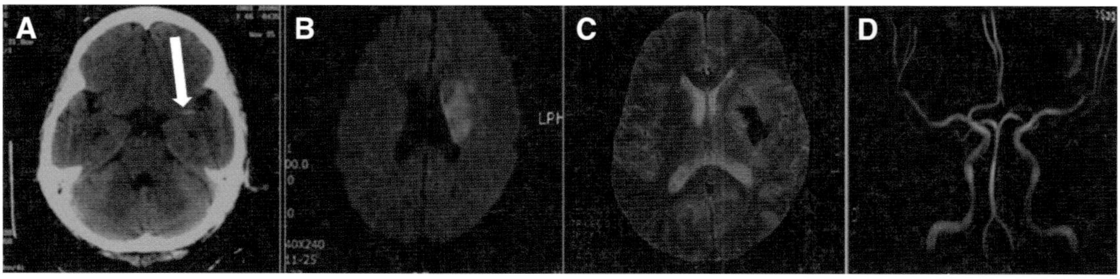

Brain CT (A) showed a dense MCA sign in the left (arrow). Brain MR-DWI (B) showed acute infarcts in the left MCA territory involving left basal ganglia, and frontal subcortical white matters. This lesion was combined with hemorrhagic transformation in the left basal ganglia (C). Brain MRA (D) showed a recanalization of the occluded left proximal MCA shown in the previous CT, but decreased vascularity of distal MCA branches, suggesting residual occlusions of distal branches. She was initially treated with antiplatelet agent because of hemorrhage transformation, and later changed with anticoagulation. Her neurologic symptoms were slowly improved.

She was diagnosed as a left middle cerebral territory multiple infarcts with hemorrhagic transformation. The mechanism of infarction was thought to be cardioembolic infarction associated with atrial fibrillation. Initial brain CT showed a dense MCA sign in the left side, but followed MRA showed a recanalization.

• Case 75

A 74-year-old woman was admitted because of a left-sided weakness, which occurred 1 day ago. Since 7 years before admission, she had suffered from atrial fibrillation and mitral stenosis, and taken digoxin. She had no history of hypertension, diabetes mellitus or previous stroke. On exam, she was alert but abulic. There was no neglect on the left side. Cranial nerve examinations were normal except for mild dysarthria. Her left limb was weak (MRC grade IV). Sensory examination showed no abnormalities to all modalities. Atrial fibrillation was noted on ECG. Echocardiography revealed left atrium enlargement without thrombi.

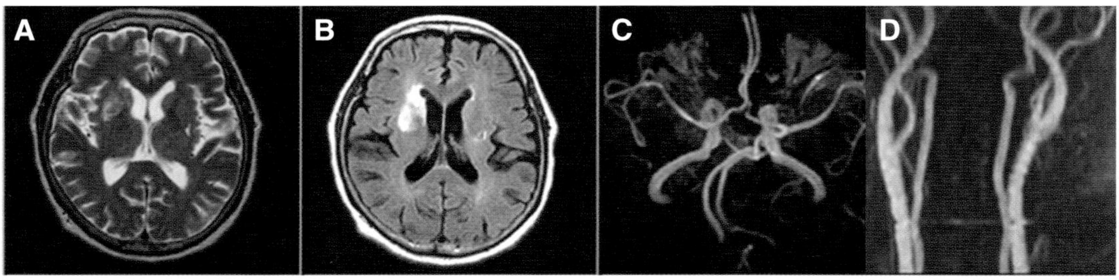

MRI (A, B) showed a right striatocapsular infarction involving the caudate head. Brain MRA (C, D) showed no definite stenosis or occlusion in the intracranial and extracranial arteries. She was treated with anticoagulant.

Striatocapsular infarction is commonly associated with cardioembolism or artery to artery embolism. In this case, the stroke mechanism was a cardioembolism.

• Case 76

A 60-year-old right-handed man was admitted because of a sudden right-sided weakness and language disturbance for 3 hours. 2 years before admission, he had suffered from atrial fibrillation and mitral stenosis. He had no history of hypertension, diabetes mellitus or previous stroke. He was slightly drowsy. Language function test showed motor aphasia with relatively possible communication. He showed the left gaze preponderance. His right limb was weak (MRC scale I). Sensory examination showed right hypesthesia to all modalities. Echocardiography revealed left atrium enlargement with thrombi and severe mitral stenosis.

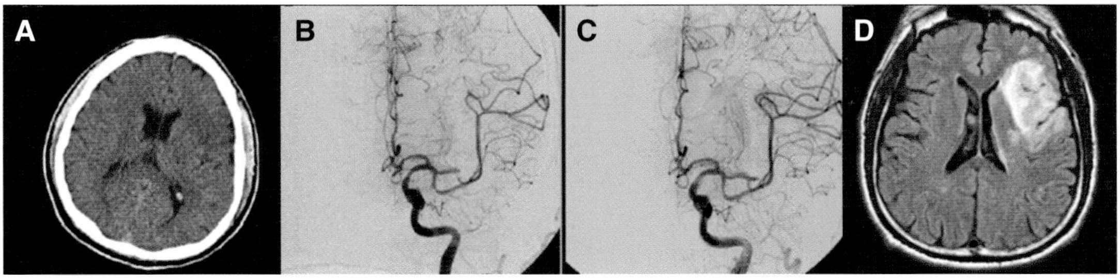

Brain CT (A) at 4 hours after symptom onset showed slightly low attenuation in the left frontal lobe. Left M1 occlusion was seen in initial evaluation (B). Intraarterial thrombolysis was done at 5 hours after symptom onset, and thereafter the partial recanalization of this artery was noted (C). Brain MR imaging (D) at 2 days after thrombolysis showed a left MCA infarction, mainly in the superior divisional area. His neurological symptoms were improved after the thrombolysis (from NIHSS 18 to 11). Thereafter, he was treated with anticoagulants. 1 month after the stroke, mitral vavuloplasty was done.

The stroke mechanism was a cardioembolism.

• Case 77

A 54-year-old right-handed man visited our hospital because of a sudden language disturbance and right-sided weakness. 2 years before admission, he had suffered from atrial fibrillation and mitral stenosis and taken digoxin. He also had a history of hypertension. He had no history of diabetes mellitus or previous stroke. He was alert. Language function test revealed sensory aphasia. He showed no gaze preponderance and visual field defect. He had a right facial weakness. His right extremities were weak (MRC grade II). Atrial fibrillation was noted on ECG. Echocardiography revealed severe mitral stenosis but no thrombi or regional wall motion abnormality.

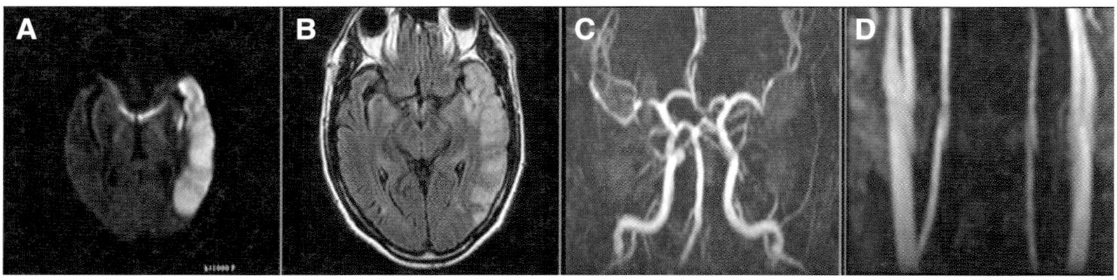

MRI (A, B) showed an acute infarction mainly involving the inferior divisional area of the left MCA. Brain MRA (C, D) showed an occlusion of the inferior branch of left MCA. Other vessels were intact. He was treated with an anticoagulant.

He had mitral stenosis and atrial fibrillation. The stroke mechanism was thought to be a cardioembolism.

• Case 78

A 69-year-old woman was hospitalized because of recurrent loss of consciousness. She had experienced loss of consciousness three times before admission. The duration of loss of consciousness was about 3 to 5 minutes. After the last event, vertical diplopia was present for about an hour. There had been a right-sided weakness due to previous stroke diagnosed 6 years prior to the admission. She had diabetes mellitus, hypertension, coronary heart disease and atrial fibrillation. She was alert and orientation was intact. Her head tilted to the right and mild weakness of right limb was also detected. There was no limb ataxia but her gait showed axial lateropulsion to the right side. Old inferior wall infarct was detected on ECG and atrial fibrillation was present. However, echocardiography showed no abnormality. FBS/HbA1c was normal.

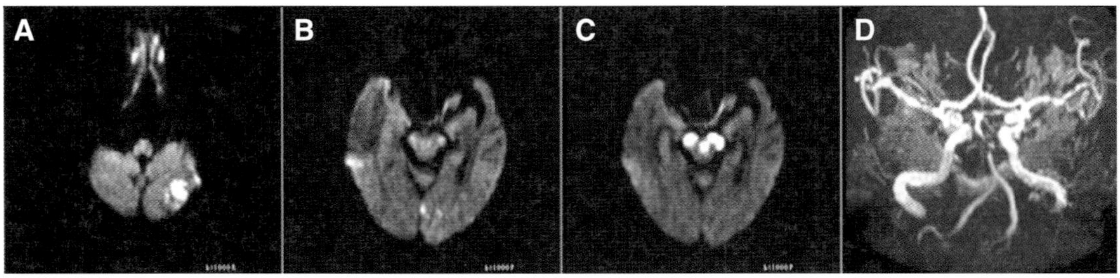

Brain MR-DWI (A, B) showed multifocal acute infarcts in the left cerebellum, posterior occiput and thalamus. She was treated with anticoagulant. In spite of that, there were recurrent transient ischemic attacks three times a week. On the tenth hospital day, new neurological defects including dysarthria and left-sided weakness developed. Follow-up DWI (C) identified new infarctions in the midbrain. Brain MRA (D) revealed a segmental narrowing of the BA and slight narrowing of the right distal ICA and bilateral proximal MCAs.

She had atrial fibrillation, acute myocardial infarction history, and recurrent stroke. There was an old infarction involving right frontal cortex. Although there were occipital and midbrain infarctions associated with a tight BA stenosis in MRA, the stroke mechanism was thought to be a cardiogenic embolism because of a simultaneous left PICA infarction.

• Case 79

A 68-year-old right handed woman developed sudden language disturbance during the usual daytime activity. At the same time, she presented a right-sided weakness. She visited a local emergency department in 4 hours. She had a history of hypertension and had regular medications. Examination showed motor aphasia without comprehension difficulty. She showed a right-sided weakness (motor MRC grade IV), but intact sensory perception in all limbs. Hyperreflexia was absent. She was able to walk in a very short distance. Initial NIHSS was 4. Transthoracic echocardiography and transesophageal echocardiography showed dilated left atrium. Holter monitoring revealed paroxysmal atrial fibrillation.

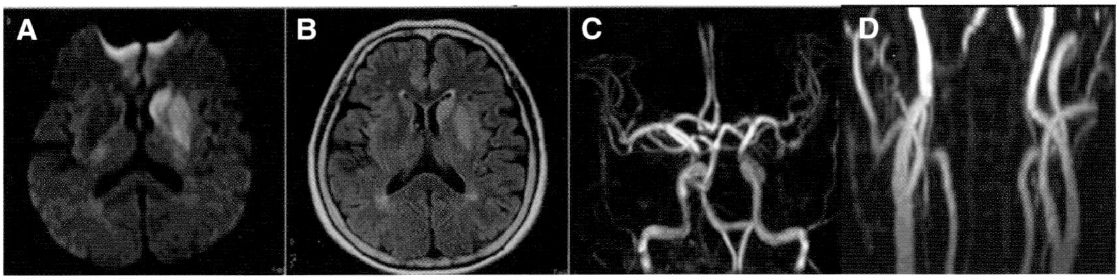

Brain MR-DWI and Flair image (A, B) showed a left striatocapsular infarction involving the caudate head. Intravenous urokinase was infused with 300,000 unit bolus injection followed by 1,500,000 unit continuous infusion for 6 hours. Brain MRA (C, D) showed no significant stenoocclusive lesions. Her symptoms were slowly improved in the next few days and could walk without assistance. Her language disturbance continued to improve. No cardiogenic embolic source was found except paroxysmal atrial fibrillation. NIHSS at discharge was 2.

The high signal intensity seen in the right striatocapsular area without MRA abnormality seemed to indicate an early recanalization of the left MCA. Considering that the distal MCA territory was also saved from the ischemia, it is possible that an embolus transiently lodged in the left MCA stem and resolved rapidly. The recanalization could happen even before the administration of urokinase. Normal MCA vasculature seen in MRA also supports this postulation.

• Case 80

A 68-year-old right handed man presented with a sudden language disturbance and left-sided weakness 1 hour before visiting the emergency department. He showed difficulty in both word fluency and comprehension. He had a history of atrial fibrillation, but had not been treated. Examination showed global aphasia, and the right central facial palsy. Strength in his right-sided limbs was MRC grade III. Diminished sensory perception in his right hemibody was evident. Hyperreflexia and Babinski sign in his right side were also present. NIHSS at admission was 19. Transthoracic echocardiography and Holter monitoring did not reveal any cardiac source of embolism.

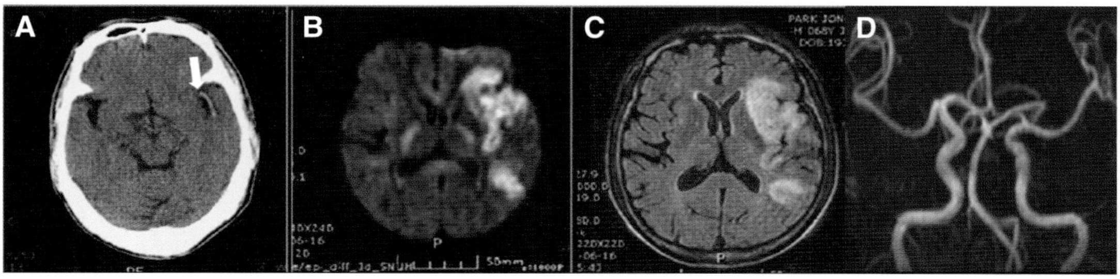

Brain CT (A) showed dense MCA sign in the left distal M1 portion (arrow). Intravenous rt-PA was administered at 2 hours after the symptom onset. MRI (B, C) showed left MCA territory acute infarction. In figure (C), here again the increased T2 change limited along the cortical mantle which suggest rapid re-supply of blood flow to the possible infracted area through the recanalization. Brain MRA (D) showed no significant stenoocclusive lesions. His global aphasia and right-sided weakness improved immediately after thrombolysis and continued to improve during the next few days. And finally, minimal neurologic deficit remained. He was discharged with warfarin medication. NIHSS at discharge was 2.

Initial Brain CT shows "Dense MCA sign" in the distal left MCA, sparing proximal portion. Considering his cadioembolic risk factor, atrial fibrillation, emboli might be plunged in the left MCA distal M1 portion. Consequently, left striatum could be saved from the ischemia. Distal MCA occlusion by embolism often recanalizes spontaneously.

• Case 81

A 76-year-old man visited our hospital because of a sudden visual disturbance and headache for 2 days. There were no motor or sensory symptoms. 10 years before admission, he had suffered from myocardial infarction. 2 years before, he had had a left MCA infarction, which resulted in a right-sided weakness. He had taken antiplatelets. He also had history of hypertension. On examination, he was slightly drowsy and showed right homonymous hemianopsia. Pure word blindness was noted on higher cortical function test. Gerstmann features were not definite. Other cranial nerve examinations were normal. Motor and sensory examination showed no abnormal findings. Echocardiography revealed lateral wall hypokinesia.

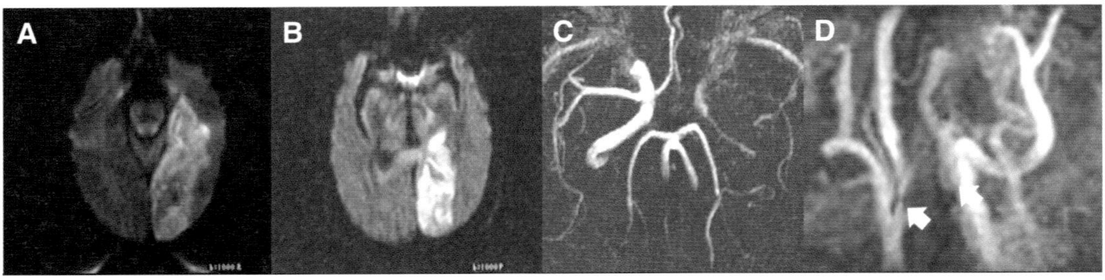

Brain MR-DWI (A, B) showed a left PCA infarct with hemorrhagic transformation. Brain MRA (C, D) showed a near occlusion of the left proximal ICA and severe stenosis of the right proximal ICA. Posterior circulation was intact at least in MRA. Antiplatelets were initially maintained because of hemorrhagic transformation, and thereafter oral anticoagulant was instituted.

In usual right handed person, the left occipital infarction with involvement of the left splenium is the typical lesion combination in pure word blindness (alexia without agraphia), a kind of disconnection syndrome. Although we did not evaluate proximal VA or aortic arch, the stroke mechanism seemed to be a cardioembolism resulting from the involving site (PCA territory) and significant regional wall motion abnormality in echocardiography.

• Case 82

A 68-year-old man presented with diplopia suddenly developed 30 minutes prior to visit when he had been driving a car. He had a hypertension and coronary heart disease. Neurologic examination showed internuclear ophthalmoplegia on the left associated with ocular tilt reaction (head tilt to the right) and skew deviation. Also central-type facial palsy on the left side and dysarthria were present. Motor power was MRC grade IV on the left hemibody. In echocardiography, apical wall akinesia due to old myocardial infarction was detected.

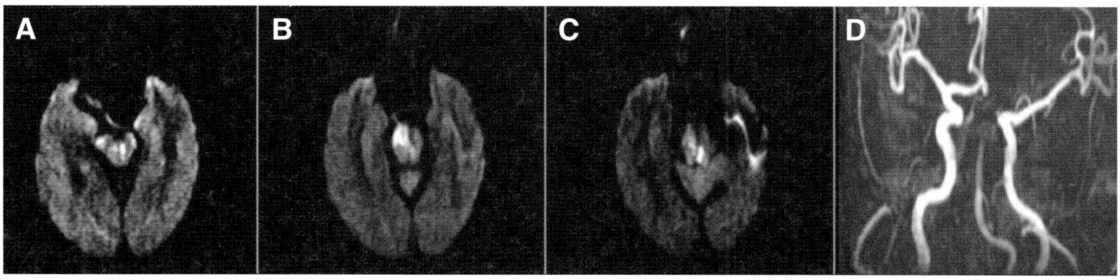

Brain MR-DWI (A-C) showed acute infarctions in the tegmentum of midbrain and pons dominantly involving right paramedian basis pontis. Brain MRA (D) showed a significant distal BA stenosis. He was treated with anticoagulant. Left hemiparesis was improved, but internuclear ophthalmoplegia persisted. Transcranial Doppler, which was performed at the time of discharge, revealed a normal flow velocity in the BA.

The mechanism of stroke was thought to be a cardioembolism to the distal BA because of initial BA stenosis in MRA and normal flow velocity later on TCD. Ocular tilt reaction, contraversive in this case, resulted from the lesion on the left midbrain and pons which involves medial longitudinal fasciculus and interstitial nucleus of Cajal, a well known integration center for eye-head coordination in roll plane.[17]

• Case 83

A 61-year-old right-handed man visited us because of a sudden right-sided weakness with ipsilateral tingling sensation. He also complained of visual disturbance. 5 years before the admission, he had suffered from hypertension and atrial fibrillation. Although he had taken regular antihypertensive drugs and digoxin, he had had a complication of chronic renal failure. He was alert. Language function test showed no abnormal findings. Visual field examination showed right upper quadrantanopsia. Motor and sensory examinations showed right-sided weakness (MRC grade IV+) and hypesthesia. Atrial fibrillation was noted on ECG. Echocardiography revealed dilated left atrium and global hypokinesia.

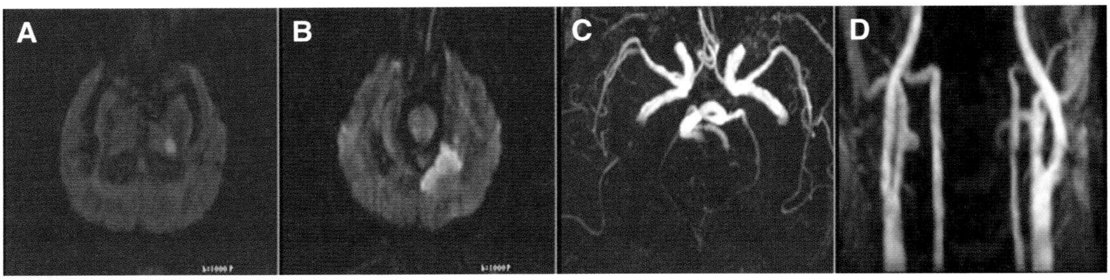

Brain MR-DWI (A, B) showed multiple infarcts in the left PCA territory. Brain MRA (C, D) showed no significant stenoocclusive lesions. He was treated with anticoagulant.

Two distinct lesions in the left thalamus and medial temporal area were located in the PCA territory. The stroke mechanism was a cardioembolism by atrial fibrillation and global hypokinesia.

• Case 84

A 52-year-old right handed man developed a right-sided weakness and aphasia 1 hour ago. He could not received intravenous rt-PA because of low platelet count (< 100,000/uL). 20 years before, he had undertaken open heart surgery due to Ebstein anomaly. He showed global aphasia of sensory-dominant type and right-sided weakness (MRC grade IV). Transesophageal echocardiography showed Ebstein anomaly, small right-to-left shunt, and dilated left atrium with severe spontaneous echogenic contrast. Abdomen ultrasonography showed hepatic congestion and mild splenomegaly.

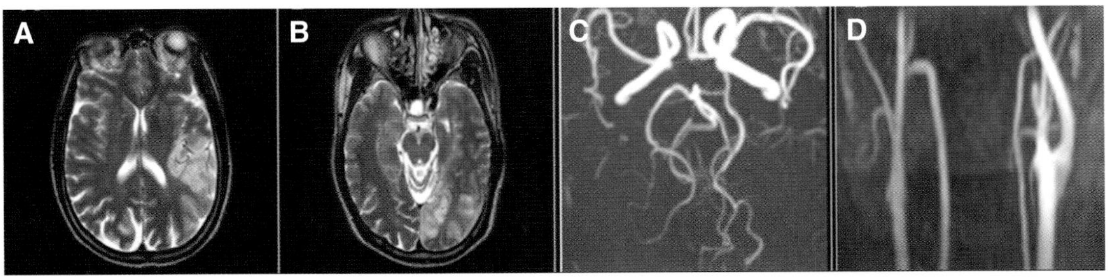

MRI (A, B) showed high signal intensity in the left MCA and PCA territory. Brain MRA (C, D) showed no significant stenosis but left PCA fetal circulation. Anticoagulation was applied to him. His weakness was much improved and sensory-dominant aphasia was slightly improved. He was discharged with warfarin medication.

The stroke mechanism was a cardioembolism to the left MCA and PCA territory through Pcom because of the dominant fetal circulation of the left PCA.

• Case 85

A 70-year-old right-handed man developed a sudden right-sided weakness and drowsiness during talking with his family members. In 1 hour, he visited the emergency department. He had a history of hypertension. He was a current smoker of 30 packyears. Examination showed drowsy mental status and global aphasia. Gaze preponderance was present to the left side. Central type right facial palsy was evident and the strength in his right limb were MRC grade II. Sensory perception in his right hemibody was also diminished. Hyperreflexia and Babinski sign was noted in his right side. Initial NIHSS was 27. Transthoracic echocardiography showed no abnormality and transesophageal echocardiography showed spontaneous echogenic contrast in left atrial appendage.

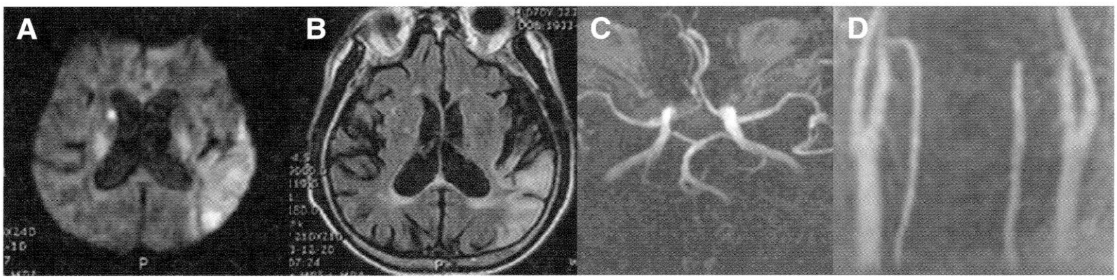

MRI showed acute multiple infarctions in the left MCA inferior division territory and right MCA perforator zone in DWI (A) and FLAIR image (B). Brain MRA (C, D) showed no significant stenoocclusive lesions. Intravenous rt-PA was tried in this patient, and there was no remarkable incident response to the thrombolysis therapy. He continued to show global aphasia and right hemiparesis. NIHSS was 18 at discharge.

Bilateral lesions involving left MCA territory and right corona radiata suggested a cardioembolism in this patient. Concomitantly, Brain MRA showed no abnormality and transesophageal echocardiography showed some evidence of cardioembolic source. Recanalization might be achieved spontaneously or by the thrombolysis without definite clinical improvement.

• Case 86

A 54-year-old right-handed woman was admitted because of a left-sided weakness and altered mentality. Since 2 years before admission, she had suffered from atrial fibrillation and mitral stenosis. She had no history of hypertension, diabetes mellitus or previous stroke. She was alert but with anosognosia. There was visual neglect on the left side. Cranial nerve examinations were normal except for mild dysarthria. Her left limb was weak (MRC grade III). Sensory examination showed left hypesthesia to all modalities. Echocardiography revealed left atrium enlargement and thrombi in the left atrium appendage.

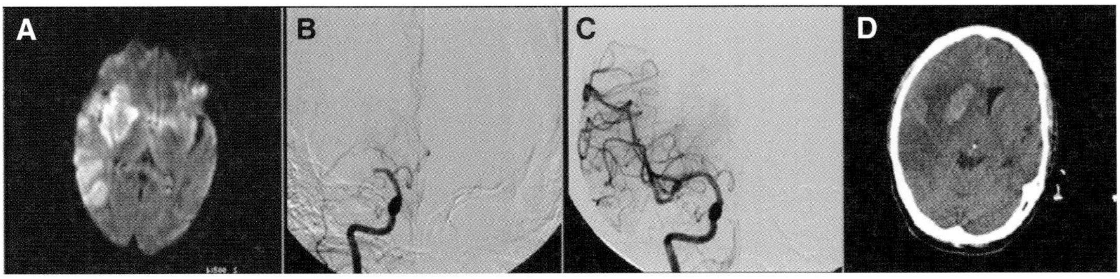

Brain MR-DWI (A) showed right MCA infarct involving penetrator and pial zones. Right M1 occlusion was seen in initial angiographic evaluation (B). Intraarterial thrombolysis was done at 4 hours after symptom onset, and thereafter the partial recannalization of the artery was noted (C). Hemorrhagic transformation was detected on follow-up brain CT (D). Her neurological symptoms were not changed in spite of thrombolysis. Thereafter, she was treated with anticoagulants.

She had mitral stenosis and atrial fibrillation. The stroke mechanism was a cardioembolism.

• Case 87

A 41-year-old man presented with a dysarthria. His past medical history did not include hypertension or diabetes mellitus. 1 day before admission, he had felt dysarthria suddenly. He did not complain any weakness or numbness. On neurologic examination, he revealed mild dysarthria and suspicious motor aphasia. Echocardiography revealed only small PFO. Holter monitoring was normal sinus rhythm.

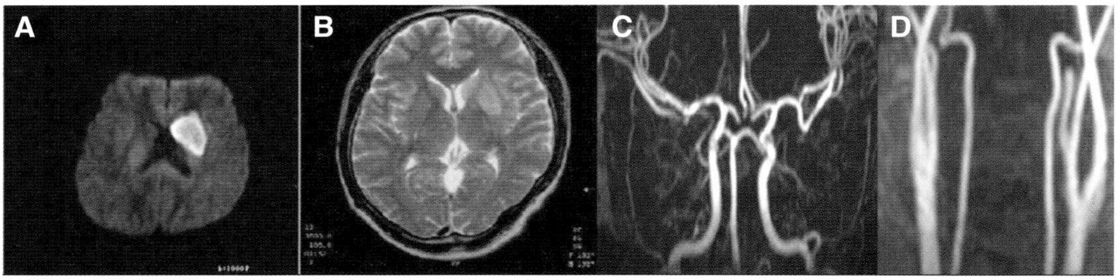

Brain MRI (A, B) showed acute infarct in left caudate and basal ganglia. Brain MRA (C, D) showed no significant stenosis in the intracranial and extracranial cerebral arteries. His symptoms were improved with antiplatelet agent therapy.

He was a young-age stroke patient. During the risk factor evaluation, small PFO was detected in transesophageal echocardiography and brain MRA showed a recanalization state of the MCA. The mechanism of stroke was presumed to be a cardioembolism to the MCA stem and resolved rapidly before the MRA examination.

• Case 88

A 69-year-old woman had been admitted to our hospital due to recurrent left-sided weakness 3 years ago. She had had medication with clopidogrel since previous recurrent TIA. She had no past medical history. 2 days ago, she showed a mental deterioration. She showed decreased verbal output and abulia. She showed mild dysphagia and decreased verbal output. Motor and sensory change was not developed. Transesophageal echocardiography showed PFO.

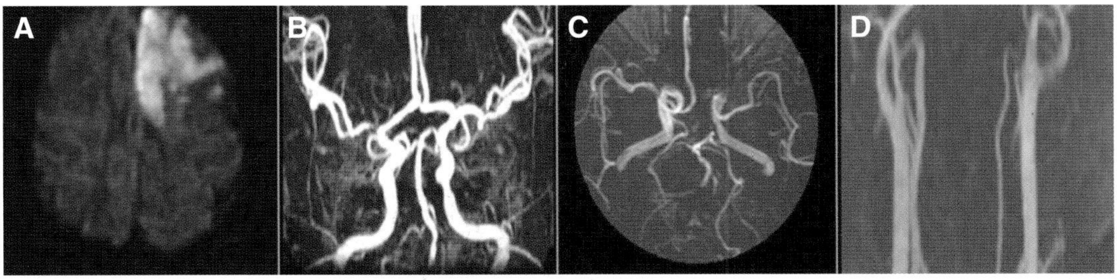

Brain MR-DWI (A) showed an acute infarction in the left ACA territory. Left ACA was normal by the MRA taken 3 years ago (B). At this admission, brain MRA (C, D) revealed left A1 occlusion and left M2 focal stenosis. After admission, anticoagulation was started. On 11th hospital day, seizure was developed. She took phenytoin intravenously and seizure was controlled.

The patient has no vascular risk factor or cardioembolic source, except PFO. The left ACA was absolutely normal 3 years ago (B), but recently the left ACA was not visualized (C). The stroke mechanism could be a cardioembolism to the left ACA.

• Case 89

A 37-year-old woman was hospitalized because of acute visual disturbance, which was developed 1 week ago. Her past medical history included migraine without aura. But there was no headache or aura accompanied with occurrence of her visual symptom. She had no risk factors of stroke. Neurologic examination revealed no abnormal findings except left upper quadrant anopsia. Transthoracic echocardiography was normal but transesophageal echocardiography showed positive result of PFO test.

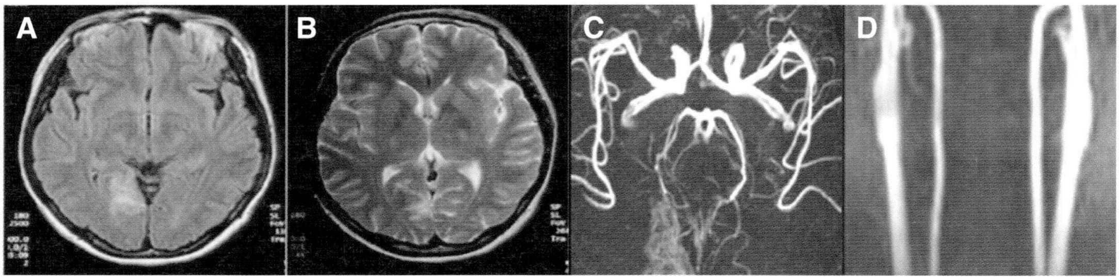

MRI (A, B) showed right PCA territory infarction. Brain MRA (C, D) showed no significant stenoocclusive lesions except mild distal PCA stenosis. She was treated with antiplatelet agent. Her visual symptom was not improved.

This is a case of a young woman migraineur who had ischemic infarction of the PCA territory. PFO test was positive but there was no stroke risk factor. Mechanism was a probably cardioembolism. These findings correspond with the characteristics of acute ischemic stroke in patients with migraine which was reported previously. However, the diagnosis of migrainous infarction was less possible because it usually occurs in patients with migraine with aura, which persists beyond 1 hour.[18]

• Case 90

A 56-year-old man visited our hospital complaining of a sudden left-sided numbness. Mild left-sided weakness was also complained of. He had an operation history for abdominal aortic aneurysm and hypertension history with regular medication. Diabetes mellitus, heart disease and hypercholesterolemia were denied. He quit smoking 6 months before but had a smoking history of 40 packyears. On visiting hospital, BP was 110/80mmHg. Mental state was alert and oriented. Cranial nerve examination and motor power were normal. Sensory examination revealed hypesthesia of 80% in the left hemibody. Deep tendon reflex was normoactive. Serum laboratory results and ECG were normal. Transthoracic echocardiography was normal but transesophageal echocardiography revealed large PFO with right to left shunt.

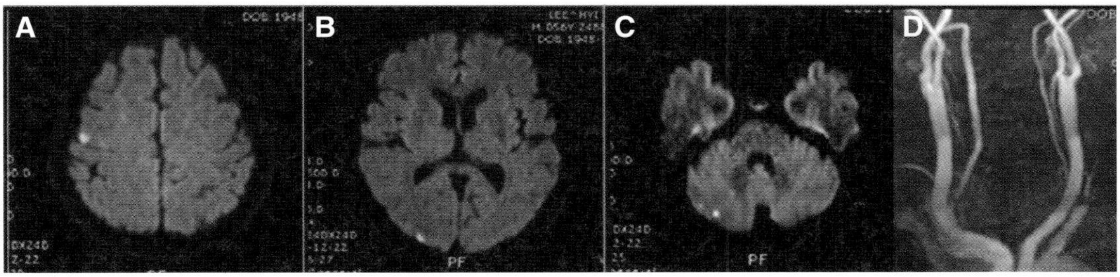

Brain MR-DWI (A-C) showed small multiple acute ischemic infarctions in the right frontal cortex, right parietooccipital cortex and right cerebellum. Brain MRA (D) showed no significant stenoocclusive lesions. He was treated with antiplatelet agent and symptoms were fully recovered.

The mechanism of stroke was thought to be a cardioembolic infarction from the large PFO.

• Case 91

A 27-year-old man came to our hospital for a sudden left-sided weakness. He was generally in good healthy through his whole life, and teacher in physical education. 1 day prior to admission, he experienced a sudden headache in the right temporal area accompanied by limb weakness and facial palsy on the left. The symptoms occurred in the course of walking, but all of the symptoms disappeared 30 minutes later. There was no abnormal finding in physical examination. Neurologic examination was entirely normal, and carotid bruit was inaudible. Echocardiography and Holter monitoring could not detect any embolic source such as left atrium thrombi or PFO. There was no abnormal finding in transcranial Doppler. Chest CT could not find any evidence of pulmonary AVM or AV fistula, either.

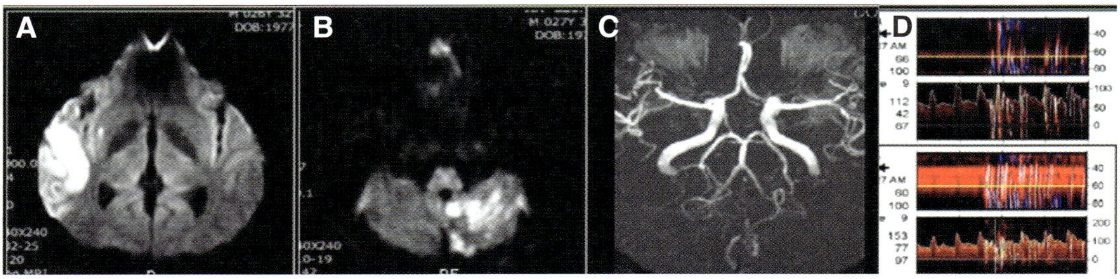

Brain MR-DWI (A) showed acute infarction in the right basal ganglia, and right temporoparietal lobe. While he was treated with anticoagulation, he revisited emergency room for a sudden vertigo and vomiting 6 months later. Neurologic examination revealed gaze paretic nystagmus and veering tendency to the left side. The initial PT-INR was 1.08 and brain MRI showed newly developed left PICA infarction (B). The symptoms were subsided the next day. Brain MRA (C) showed no significant stenoocclusive lesions. Transcranial doppler detected microembolic signal on the agitated saline test with Valsalva maneuver (D). Transesophageal echocardiography also detected PFO in this time.

The stroke mechanism was a cardioembolism by PFO in this case. In the first attack, the saline agitation test during the TCD was not done in belief of negative PFO result on transesophageal echocardiography. In addition, patients often might not do Valsalva maneuver well during the TEE or TCD examination for PFO detection. The two tests are supplementary, not competing in detection of PFO. TCD with saline test is reported to be more sensitive test for a minimal right-to-left shunt.[19]

3. Small Vessel Occlusion

• Case 92

A 46-year-old man was admitted due to the right-sided weakness developed 2 days ago. 3 days before admission, he had developed transient right lower extremity weakness. He denied all risk factors except alcohol drinking. He showed right-sided weakness (MRC grade IV), right-sided ataxia and veering to the right. Fundus examination showed hypertensive retinopathy grade II-III. Transthoracic echocardiography and Holter monitoring did not reveal any cardiac source of embolism.

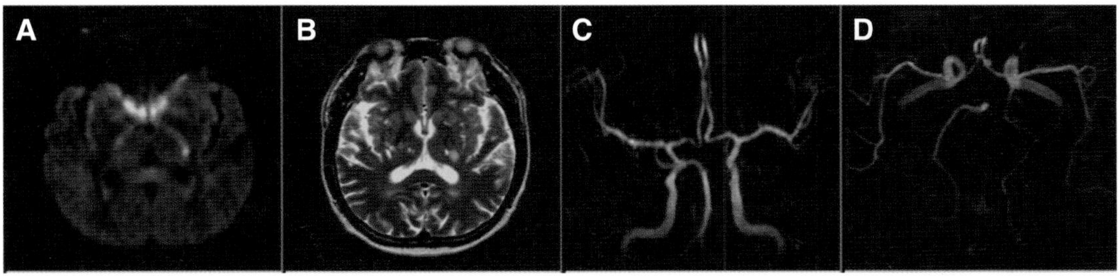

Brain MR-DWI (A) showed a left internal capsule infarction. T2WI (B) showed multiple high signal intensities in the left internal capsule lesion and bilateral periventricular white matter lesion. Brain MRA (C, D) showed no significant stenoocclusive lesions. We started antiplatelet. His neurological symptom was improved.

The lacunar syndrome of this case was ataxic hemiparesis. His symptom was due to left internal capsule lesion abutting ventral postero-lateral nucleus of thalamus. He was newly diagnosed to have a hypertension. Multiple small deep infarct and retinopathy were evidences of his chronic hypertension.

• Case 93

A 45-year-old man was admitted because of sudden right-sided weakness. 3 years before admission, he had suffered from hypercholesterolemia but with irregular medication. He had no history of hypertension, heart disease or previous stroke. He was alert and oriented. Language functions were intact. Cranial nerve examinations revealed mild dysarthria and right facial palsy of the central type. His right extremities were mildly weak (MRC scale IV+). Sensory examination showed no sensory loss to all modalities. Cholesterol was 277mg/dL, and HbA1C was 8.6. Echocardiography showed no remarkable abnormalities.

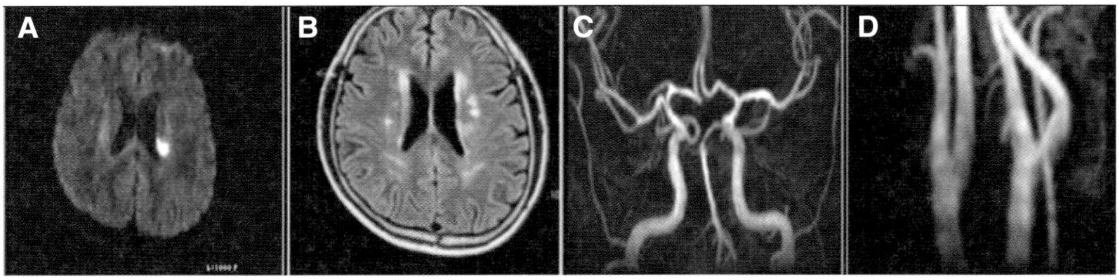

Brain MR-DWI and FLAIR (A, B) showed an acute infarct in the left corona radiata. Brain MRA (C, D) showed no significant stenoocclusive lesions. He was treated with antiplatelet agent.

He had a lacunar syndrome of pure motor hemiparesis resulting from corona radiata lesion. The stroke mechanism was a small vessel occlusion.

• Case 94

A 71-year-old man, right-handed presented with a sudden onset of left-sided weakness, which was developed 1 day prior to visit. He had been diagnosed as vascular dementia 2 years before and left corona radiata infarction resulting in right-sided weakness 1 year before. He had a hypertension. His medication included galantamine and triflusal. He was alert. The score of mini-mental status examination was 22. Weakness involving face and limbs on the left side was detected and graded as MRC grade III. Transthoracic echocardiography and Holter monitoring did not reveal any cardiac source of embolism.

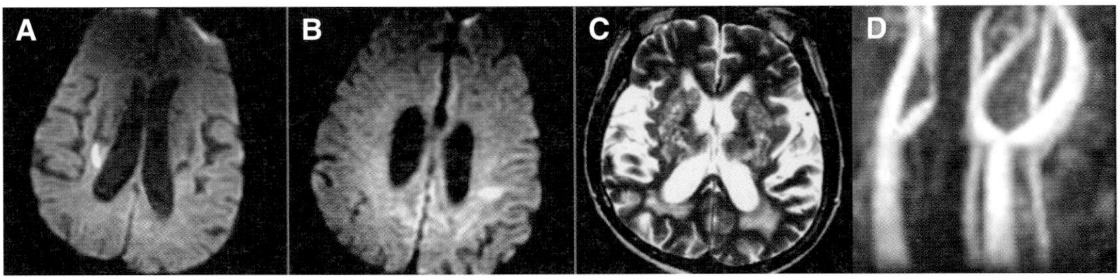

Brain MR-DWI (A, B) showed acute infarction in the right corona radiata and subacute infarction in the left corona radiate. T2WI (C) showed severe small vessel disease in the white matter, basal ganglia and thalamus. Brain MRA (D) showed a severe stenosis in the right proximal ICA. He was treated with combination of two anitplatelet agents, clopidogrel and triflusal.

MRI showed severe small vessel disease. Although there was severe stenosis in the right proximal ICA, the stroke mechanism was thought to be small vessel occlusion. Cognitive impairment and silent lesions of the deep brain structures (basal ganglia, thalamus, and white-matters) detected on MRI are often encountered in severe small vessel disease cases.

• Case 95

A 65-year-old man presented with aspiration tendency, which had occurred suddenly 2 days prior to visit. 3 years before, he had been diagnosed with multiple cerebral infarctions and vascular dementia. 2 years before, he had felt sudden vertigo and diagnosed with left lateral medullary hemorrhage. He had a long history of hypertension. His medication included triflusal and donepezil. He was disoriented to time and place. Mini-mental status examination was 11/30. Dysarthria and dysphagia were detected. Weakness was present in all four extremities. Echocardiogram showed no abnormal findings but increased left ventricular wall thickness. ApoE gene type was e3/e3.

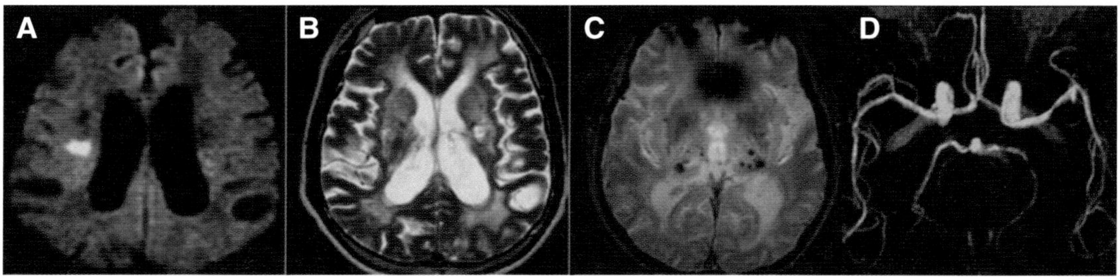

Brain MR-DWI (A) showed an acute corona radiata infarction. T2WI (B) and GRE (C) image showed diffuse ischemic lesion and multiple microbleeds with old lacunes in both hemispheres. Brain MRA (D) showed no significant lesion, except focal stenosis on the left M1 and PCA. Dysphagia was not improved. He was treated with antiplatelet agent.

There were diffuse leukoaraiosis and multiple microbleeds in the both hemispheres, the extent or number were increased on follow-up images. The stroke mechanism was thought to be a small vessel occlusion.

• Case 96

A 76-year-old man came to our hospital for a sudden left-sided weakness. He had a medical history of pituitary adenoma, but was generally in good healthy state through his life. 1 day prior to admission, he had experienced a sudden left-sided weakness in the middle of voiding. He could barely walk with cane, and the symptoms disappeared 40 minutes later. However, he experienced another attack of a left leg weakness and dysarthria after 3 hours. There were no stroke risk factors such as hypertension, diabetes mellitus, hypercholesterolemia, and smoking. Neurologic examination revealed motor weakness (MRC grade IV+) in the left leg sparing arm. He complained some decreased sense on the left limb without objective change. Echocardiography did not show any abnormal finding.

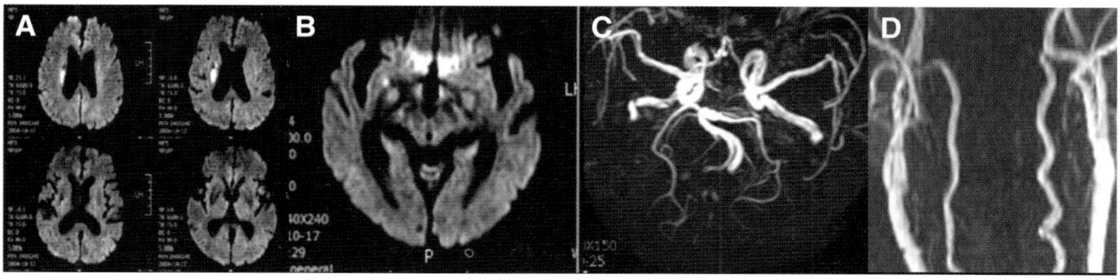

Brain MR-DWI (A, B) showed an acute infarction in the right corona radiate. Brain MRA (C, D) showed no significant stenoocclusive lesions. He was given dual antiplatelet agents (aspirin and clopidogrel). The symptoms slightly improved at discharge.

The stroke mechanism was a small vessel occlusion. The clinical manifestation of lacunar infarction in the MCA perforator occasionally might have progressive or fluctuating course. The corticospinal tracts pass the lenticulostriate artery territory exclusively at the posterosuperior quadrant, and the degree of this tract involvement within the infarcts was directly related to stroke severity and functional recovery.[20] In this case, the patient generally had more severe weakness in the leg than arm because the lesion involved the posterior part of corona radiata.

• Case 97

An 80-year-old man presented with right-sided weakness, which was developed 1 day prior to visiting hospital. He had taken clopidogrel since the previous left thalamic infarction 5 years ago. He was a current smoker of 50 packyears. However, there was no history of hypertension, and diabetes mellitus. The mental status was alert. The cranial nerve examination showed no abnormal findings except mild dysarthria. The motor power of the right side was MRC grade IV in the upper and lower extremity. The sensory examination showed a right-sided hypesthesia to the pain and temperature probably due to previous stroke. Transthoracic echocardiography and Holter monitoring did not reveal any cardiac source of embolism.

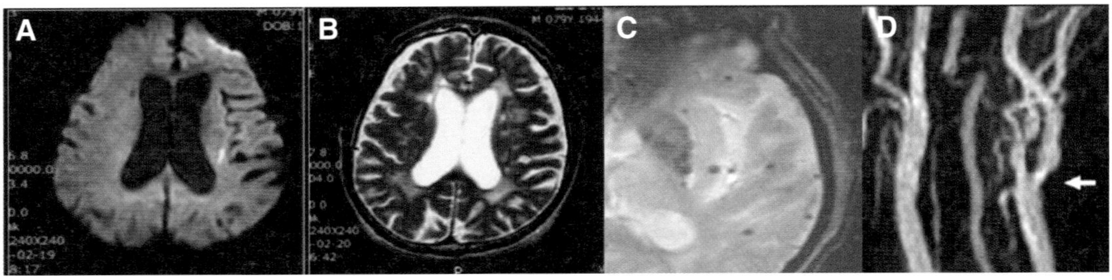

Brain MR-DWI (A) showed an acute infarction in the left periventricular white matter. T2WI (B) showed old multiple lacunes. Multiple microhemorrhages were detected in GRE image (C). Brain MRA (D) revealed a focal narrowing of the left proximal ICA (arrow), but there was no definite intracranial artery stenosis. Because new stroke was developed in spite of medication of clopidogrel, he was treated with aspirin and clopidogrel combination. His neurological symptoms improved steadily.

Although there was a focal narrowing in the left proximal ICA, the stroke mechanism was a small vessel occlusion. Microbleeds in GRE image and multiple lacunes in the basal ganglia and corona radiata are common findings owing to shared etiology of hypertension.

• Case 98

A 59-year-old woman presented with a sudden onset of the right hand weakness, which was developed 3 days prior to visit. 10 years before, she had been diagnosed with hypertension but had not taken regular medication. The ophthalmoscopic examination showed hypertensive retinopathy with grade II. Other neurologic examination revealed no abnormal findings but decreased grasping and fanning power of the right hand. Mild concentric LVH was detected on the echocardiography. The Holter monitoring showed normal findings.

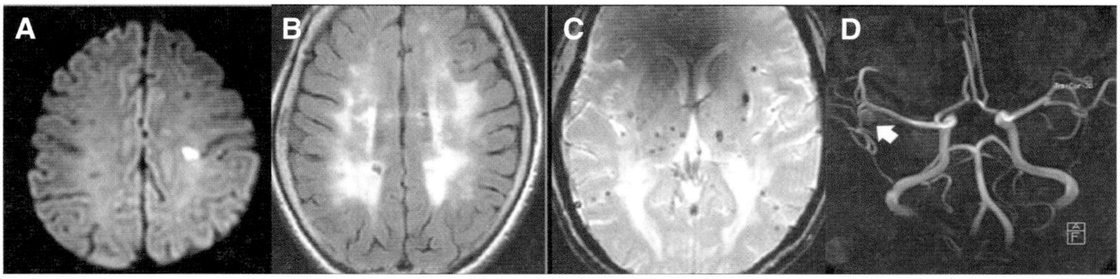

Brain MR-DWI (A) showed an acute infarction in the left frontal subcortical white matter. FLAIR image showed a severe degree of small vessel disease (B). On GRE image (C), multiple microbleeds were detected in both hemispheres. Brain MRA (D) showed no stenosis but 7mm-sized aneurysm in the right MCA bifurcation (arrow). She was treated with aspirin. She was transferred to the department of neurosurgery for the treatment of aneurysm.

There were many evidences of target organ damage resulting from uncontrolled hypertension. From the findings of diffuse leukoaraiotic change and multiple microbleeds on the MRI, she was diagnosed with hypertensive microangiopathy. Intracranial aneurysm was an incidental finding rather than hypertensive change. The stroke mechanism was thought to be a small vessel occlusion.

• Case 99

A 70-year-old right-handed man presented with sudden onset of left hemiparesis and paresthesia for 1 day. He had a history of hypertension, diabetes mellitus, and hypercholesterolemia. He had no family or previous history of stroke. Examination showed a dysarthric man complaining of pain and numbness of the left side of his body. There was no motor or visual neglect on the left side. The left upper extremity was clumsy and mildly weak (MRC grade III). Distally he had a "thalamic hand" posture. His left lower extremity was weak (MRC grade IV-) and he had an ipsilateral hemisensory loss. In particular, his proprioceptive deficit was pronounced, unable to detect up to 30 degrees of the left elbow joint movement. Transthoracic echocardiography and Holter monitoring did not reveal any cardiac source of embolism.

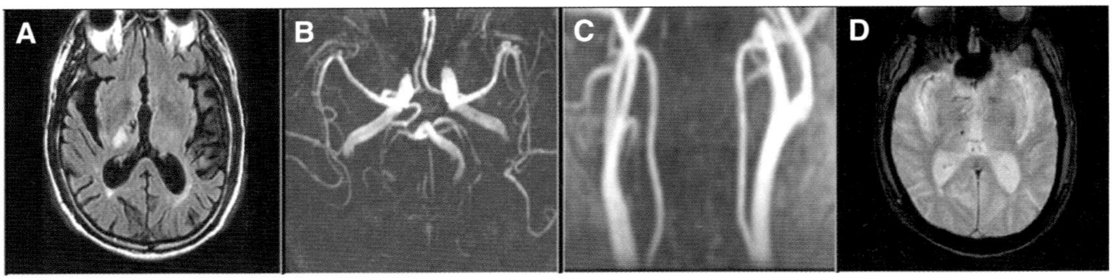

Brain FLAIR image (A) showed a right thalamic infarct. Brain MRA (B, C) showed no significant stenoocclusive lesions. We detected one small microbleed in the infarct lesion of the right medial thalamus incidentally (D). He was treated with antiplatelet agent. His neurological symptoms improved steadily.

The stroke mechanism was a small vessel occlusion. Thalamic lacunar infarction is characterized by peculiar hand posture and profound loss of proprioception.

• Case 100

A 79-year-old man came to our hospital with sudden abnormal behavior. He had past medical history of hypertension for 2 years. 3 days prior to admission, he showed abulia and apathy after taking a nap. From the next day he became angry about trivial things and said silly words. He showed mild sleeping tendency. In the mini-mental score examination, total score was 22 with a decrease in orientation (-1), serial 7 (-4), recall (-2) and interlocking pentagon (-1). Cranial nerve examination was normal except right ptosis. Other neurologic examination was all normal. ECG and echocardiography were all normal.

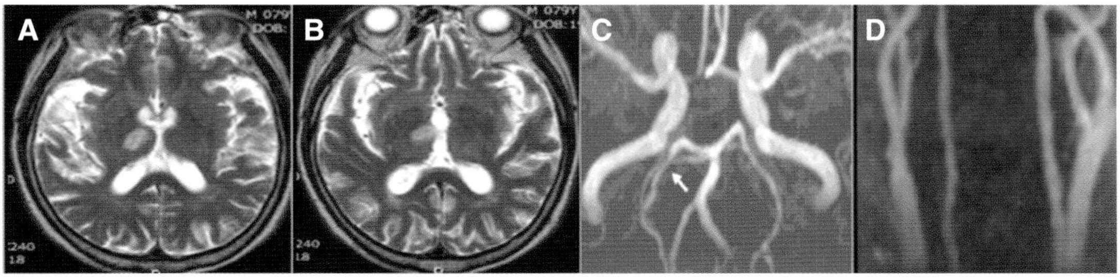

MRI (A, B) showed ischemic infarction, probably acute, 1.5cm sized in the right thalamus. Brain MRA (C, D) showed a segmental narrowing of the right proximal PCA and a mild narrowing of the right proximal ICA and ECA. He was treated with aspirin and risperidone. But, neuropsychological abnormalities persisted until discharge.

Infarcts in the territory of the paramedian thalamic arteries are the second most frequent next to lateral infarcts in the thalamus. The main etiology in this territory is embolic, but the stroke mechanism of this patient was a small vessel occlusion of the thalamic-subthalamic artery. Classic triad symptoms in the unilateral infarcts of the paramedian polar arteries are an acute decrease of consciousness, neuropsychological disturbances (unconcerned, apathetic, amnesia, confabulation) and abnormalities of vertical gaze.[21]

• Case 101

A 52-year-old woman was admitted due to a sudden memory disturbance. She had no medical history of diabetes mellitus and hypertension. She was a current smoker of 60 packyears. 7 days before admission, she couldn't remember what she had said and asked the same things repetitively. In the mini-mental status examination, total score was 26 with a decrease in memory recall (-3) and serial seven (-1). Neurologic examination revealed an impaired recent memory. However, cranial nerve examination, motor power and sensory examinations were all intact. The transthoracic echocardiography was also within normal limit.

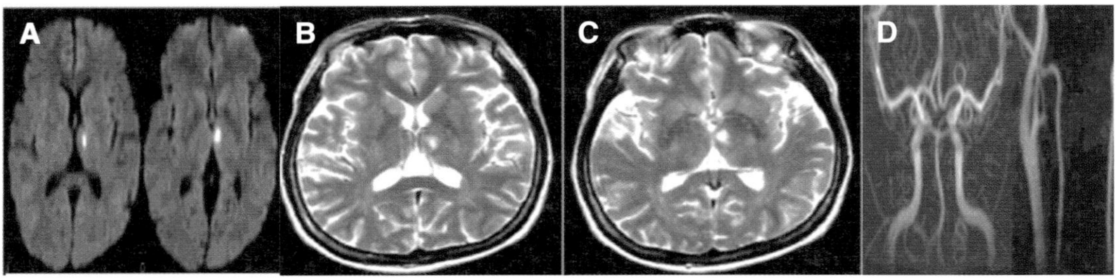

MRI (A-C) showed small acute lacunar infarct in the left anterior ventral thalamus. Brain MRA (D) revealed no abnormalities except both PCA fetal circulations. She was treated with aspirin. Her memory disturbance improved steadily. Score of memory recall at discharge was 1 (-2).

The stroke mechanism was a small vessel occlusion. After anterior (polar) infarcts, amnesia is found in combination with abulia, decreased expression of emotions, language disturbances or neglect, but a case of pure amnesia has also been described.[21] This patient also showed a pure amnesia involving memory circuit (Papez).

• Case 102

A 64-year-old woman was admitted because of sudden dysarthria. He also complained of the right hand weakens. 3 years before admission, he had suffered from hypertension and diabetes mellitus with irregular medication. She had no history of heart disease or previous stroke. She was alert and oriented. Cranial nerve examinations were normal except for mild dysarthria. Her left upper extremity was mildly weak (MRC grade IV+). Sensory examination showed no abnormal findings. Ataxia, tremor and gait abnormality were not noted. Transthoracic echocardiography and Holter monitoring did not reveal any cardiac source of embolism.

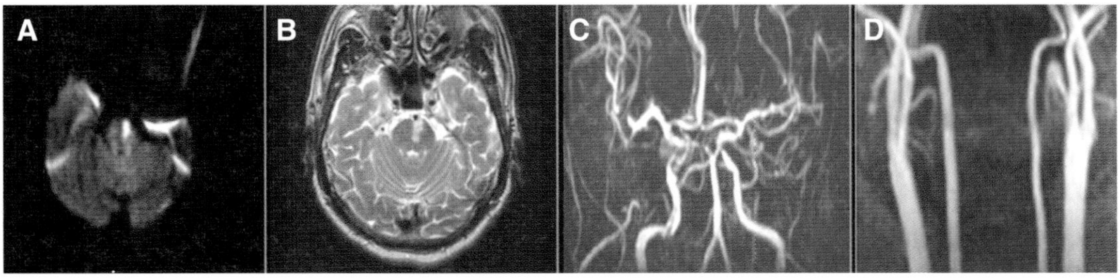

MRI (A, B) showed a left pontine infarct. Brain MRA (C, D) showed right M2 and distal ICA stenoses but with intact BA. Hypertension and diabetes mellitus were well controlled. She was treated with an antiplatelet agent.

The stroke mechanism was a small vessel occlusion. The morphology of infarction was from the base of pons, like branch atheromatous disease of pontine penetrator, but a signal void of the BA on T2WI was normal.

• Case 103

A 79-year-old man was admitted to our hospital complaining of tendency to veering rightward with a mild dizziness, which was developed 4 days ago. He did not complain of nausea and vomiting. He had a hypertension and Bell's palsy two times. Mental status was normal. Light reflex was prompt in both eyes and pupils were isocoric. There was internuclear ophthalmoplegia on the right side (limitation of right eye adduction and abducting nystagmus of the left eye) but convergence was intact. There was ataxia on the right limb and tendency to veering rightward. Motor power and sensory were intact. Transthoracic echocardiography and Holter monitoring did not reveal any cardiac source of embolism.

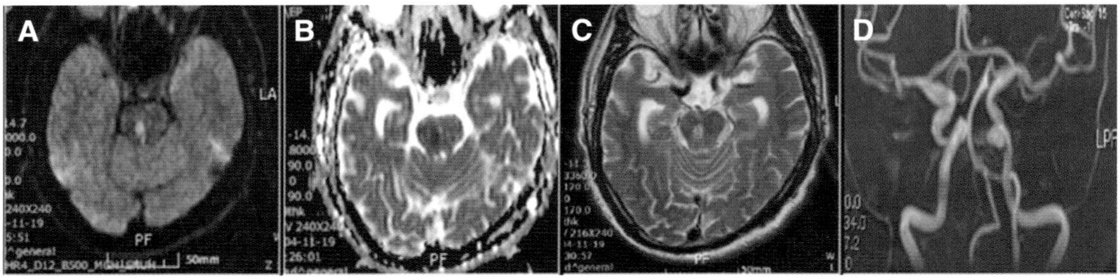

MRI (A-C) showed an acute ischemic infarct in the right paramedian pons. There were also chronic ischemic lesions on the bilateral periventricular white matter. On the brain MRA (D), there was a tortuous vertebrobasilar artery without significant stenosis and localized ectatic change in the left distal ICA. He was treated with antiplatelet agent.

The symptoms were due to an occlusion of the paramedian penetrating artery supplying corticopontocerebellar tract and medial longitudinal fasciculus. Infarcts involving only part of the tegmentum probably result from distal small penetrator occlusion.

• Case 104

A 70-year-old man presented with a sudden tingling sensation on the left side and incoordination on the day of visit. He had hypertension and hyperlipidemia with regular treatment. He was a current smoker. He had also experienced previous ischemic stroke history with left-sided weakness 2 years before. He had taken aspirin. The mental status was alert. The cranial nerve examination showed no remarkable findings. His motor power was MRC grade V. The sensory examination showed hyperesthesia 50% in proprioception on the left side. The cerebellar function test revealed dysmetria on the left side. The carotid/ophthalmic bruits were inaudible. The lipid profile was normal. The ECG and Holter monitoring were all normal.

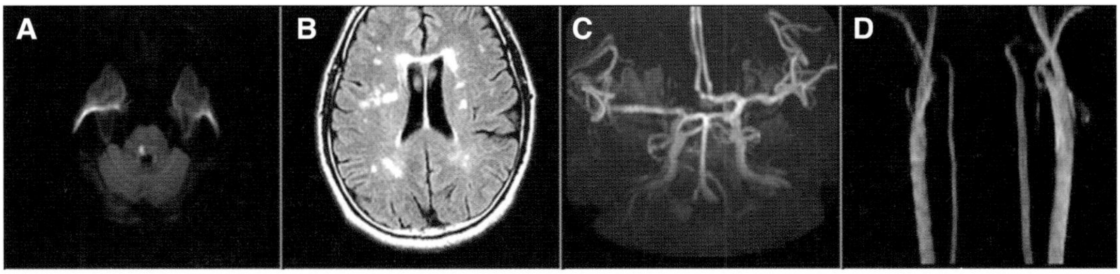

Brain MR-DWI (A) showed an acute infarction in the right pontine tegmentum. FLAIR image (B) showed moderate small vessel changes. Brain MRA (C, D) showed no significant stenoocclusive lesions. Clopidogrel was added to aspirin. His symptoms were slowly improved.

The infarction in this patient was due to an occlusion of the short penetrator of BA. The symptom in this patient was thought to result from a proprioceptive loss.

• Case 105

A 51-year-old man visited our emergency room for a right-sided weakness. He had a previous medical history of 20-year hypertension and 25-year and 15-year strokes. He didn't drink alcohol, but was a 30-pack-year current smoker. On admission day, he realized a right-sided weakness on awakening. He also felt nausea, vomiting, dysarthria and right-sided tingling sensation. His mental status was alert. Neurologic examination revealed upbeat nystagmus, right central-type facial palsy, dysarthria, and right-sided weakness (MRC grade IV). Sensory was symmetrically intact. Deep tendon reflex showed hyperactive knee jerk and Babinski sign was equivocal on the right side. The carotid bruit was inaudible. Transthoracic echocardiography and Holter monitoring did not reveal any cardiac source of embolism.

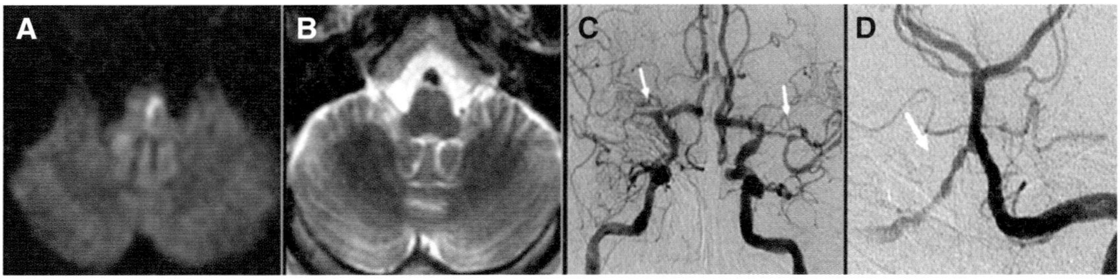

Brain MR-DWI (A) showed an acute ischemic infarction in the paramidline left medulla oblongata. T2WI (B) showed an intact signal void of left VA. Conventional angiography (C, D) showed multiple intracranial artery stenosis or occlusion including irregularity of MCA and VA (arrows). Severe stenoses of both ACAs and both MCAs, and mild stenosis of VA and BA were also detected in the transcranial Doppler. He was treated with an antiplatelet agent, and motor power was improved.

Although this patient had a diffuse intracranial atherosclerosis, the stroke mechanism was thought to be a small vessel occlusion. Patient's symptoms result from the dorsal extension of ischemic insult toward the medial longitudinal fasciculus, but the medial lemniscal system was likely to be intact because of no sensory deficits.

III

Atypical Mechanisms

• Case 106

A 44-year-old man came to our hospital for the involuntary movement of left limb that had developed 2 months ago. This attack occurred 5 to 15 times daily. The symptom duration was 5 to 10 seconds, and arm and leg was involved at the same time at all events. At the time of event, alertness and awareness were preserved, and facial muscles were spared. He had no history of hypertension, diabetes mellitus, developmental problem and head trauma. He had a mild left facial palsy, limb weakness (MRC grade IV), and dysarthria. But, the examination of sense and deep tendon reflex was normal. Mini-mental status examination was within normal limit. The carotid bruit was inaudible. The Holter monitoring and echocardiography showed no remarkable findings.

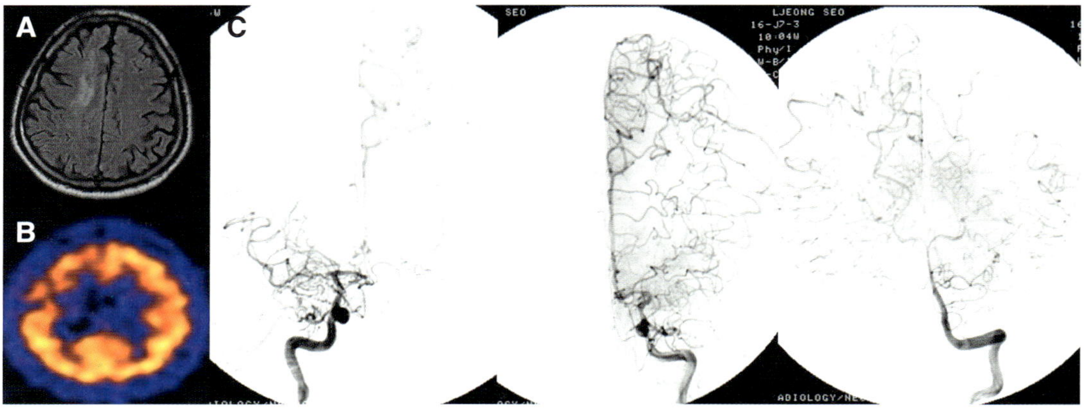

On brain FLAIR image (A), there was a subacute infarction in the right frontal area corresponding to the ACA-MCA borderzone and internal borderzone. Brain SPECT (B) showed a decreased vascular reserve in the right frontoparietal lobe. Conventional angiography (C) showed occlusions of right M1, right A2, left M1, and parietooccipital branch of left PCA, and basal collaterals. He underwent EDAS surgery. All of his symptoms disappeared after surgery.

Limb shaking in moyamoya disease may result from a transient hypoperfusion of the contralateral frontoparietal cortex rather than basal ganglia.[22] In this patient, TIA was thought to be a low flow phenomenon considering frequent attacks, significant stenoocclusive lesions, and hypoperfusion in the corresponding areas.

• Case 107

A 30-year-old man visited our hospital complaining of a sudden language disturbance. Motor and sensory symptoms were not associated. He had a stroke history of right-sided weakness. He also had a hypertension history with regular medication. His son had a similar stroke history. On visiting hospital, BP was 140/100mmHg. Mental status was alert, but Gerstmann feature was detected and language function test revealed sensory aphasia. Other neurologic exams were all normal. Serum laboratory results and ECG were normal. Transthoracic echocardiography was normal.

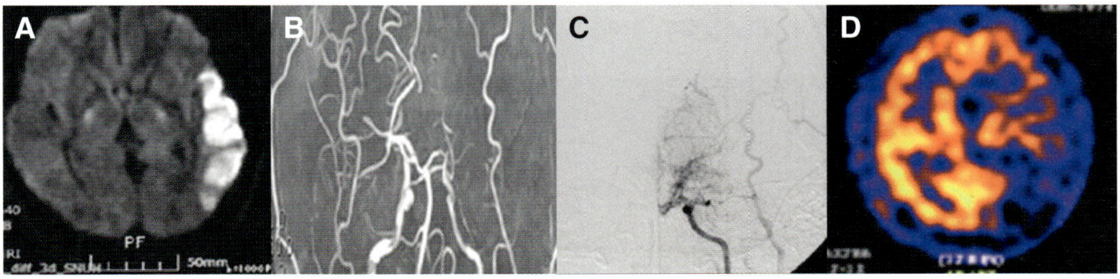

Brain MR-DWI (A) showed an acute infarct with cortical swelling in the left temporoparietal area. Brain MRA (B) showed occlusions of right MCA, left PCA, and left distal ICAs. Conventional angiography identified basal collaterals in the occluded site (C). SPECT (D) identified a perfusion defect in the left parieto-temporo-occipital lobes, and a decreased vascular reserve in the left fronto-temporo-parieto-occipital lobes He was treated with antiplatelet agent and volume expansion. His symptom was rapidly improved.

He was a moyamoya patient and had two episodes of ischemic stroke. Brain SPECT revealed a decreased vascular reserve in the left hemisphere. Bypass surgery was considered to be beneficial in this patient. Usually, ischemic strokes from moyamoya are TIA of low flow type and atypical water-shed zone infarct after transformed original vasculature.

• Case 108

A 42-year-old woman, who had had a transient right-sided weakness and hypesthesia 1 year before, was admitted due to a sudden right arm paresthesia and language disturbance. Since the episode of weakness, she had taken aspirin and antihypertensive drug. 3 days before admission, she had suddenly felt a right arm tingling sense and could not express herself. The paresthesia had been recovered in 1 hour after onset, but the language disturbance was not improved till admission. Her fluency and naming was much impaired, but repetition and comprehension was preserved. Neurologic examination did not reveal any motor or sensory change. In laboratory tests, abnormal findings were not observed. ECG and echocardiography were normal.

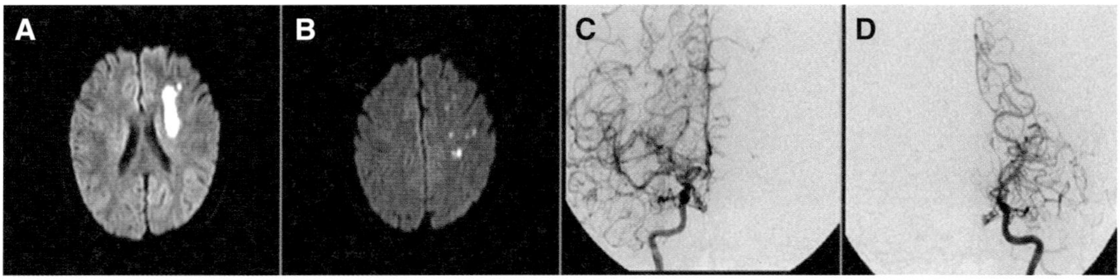

Brain MR-DWI (A, B) showed acute infarctions in the left subcortex and basal ganglia. Conventional angiography (C, D) showed bilateral distal ICA occlusions with multichannel collaterals. The language symptom of transcortical motor aphasia was slightly improved. She was discharged with medication of aspirin and clopidogrel. She was supposed to be operated for EDAS surgery in other hospital.

Bilateral MCAs were not visualized in her TFCA being compatible with moyamoya disease. The patient has recurrent cerebral ischemic symptoms, which may be due to impaired cerebral perfusion. Transcortical motor aphasia resulted from lesion in the frontal subcortical area. The infarction was due to a hypoperfusion of atypical watershed zone of the left MCA. EDAS would be needed for preventing further ischemic events.

• Case 109

A 41-year-old man was admitted because of a sudden left-sided weakness. 3 weeks before admission, he had taken scaling service at the dental clinic, and thereafter had fever and skin rash. 1 day before, the left-sided weakness had developed suddenly. He had no history of diabetes mellitus, heart disease or previous stroke. He was slightly drowsy. There was motor or visual neglect on the left side. Right gaze preponderance was noted, and anosognosia was suspected. His left limb was weak (MRC scale III). Sensory examination showed ipsilateral sensory loss to all modalities. ECG was normal. Echocardiography showed vegetation on the mitral valve. Streptococcus viridans was demonstrated from blood culture.

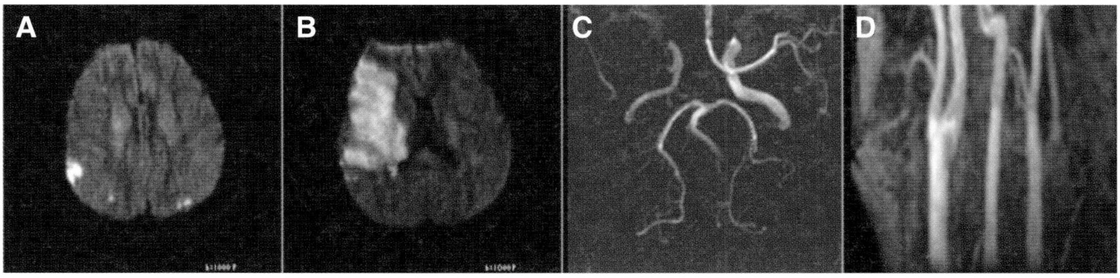

Brain MR-DWI (A, B) showed multiple lesions in the right frontal and parietal areas and left parietal area. Brain MRA (C, D) showed an occlusion in the right distal ICA and no stenosis in the neck vessels. He was treated with antibiotics and antiplatelet agent. His neurological symptoms improved steadily. 6 weeks later, follow-up echocardiography was done and revealed no vegetation.

He was diagnosed as a subacute infective endocarditis with vegetation on the mitral valve. The stroke mechanism was thought to be a cardioembolism.

• Case 110

A 47-year-old, right-handed man presented with a sudden onset of aphasia, which was developed on awakening. He had experienced a left-sided weakness 3 days prior to visit but had not sought for medical advice. Aphasia was accompanied in the morning of the day when he was hospitalized. He had advanced gastric cancer with multiple metastases and was at terminal stage. He had no risk factors for stroke. He was alert, but global aphasia and left-sided weakness (MRC grade II) were detected. Mitral regurgitation murmur was audible at apex. Peripheral arterial occlusion was detected on finger tips. ECG was normal but transthoracic echocardiography revealed mild mitral regurgitation with suspected vegetation at mitral leaflet. The results of blood culture were normal. PT was slightly prolonged. FDP and d-dimer were positive.

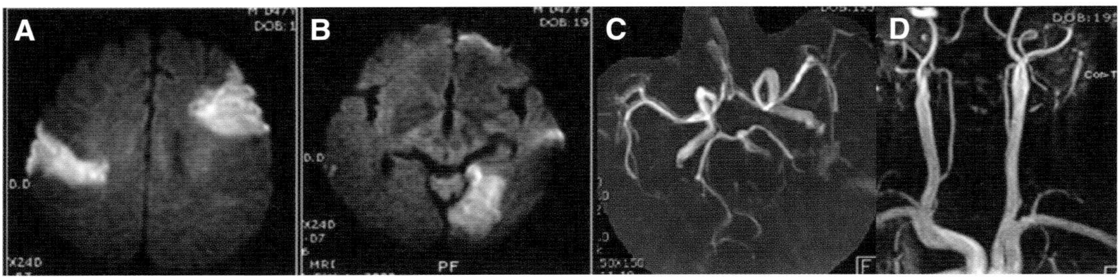

Brain MR-DWI (A, B) showed acute infarctions in both MCA territories and left PCA territories. Brain MRA (C, D) showed an occlusion of the left distal PCA and both distal MCA and normal neck angiography. He was treated with antiplatelet agent and empirical antibiotics, which were stopped due to upper gastrointestinal bleeding. He was transferred to the department of internal medicine.

Vegetations on the heart valves were suspected on echocardiography but no microogranism was identified on blood cultures. There were systemic manifestations of embolic arterial occlusion (finger tip and brain). The mechanism of stroke was thought to be a cardioembolism due to marantic endocarditis. It results from the hypercoagulable state and is characterized by uninfected vegetation in patients with malignancy or chronic disease.[23]

• Case 111

A 50-year-old woman was hospitalized because of a sudden left-sided weakness with numbness. About 1 week before, she had had a transient weakness (< 1 min., 3-4 times). She had no risk factors for stroke. She was alert and oriented. No cortical signs were detected. Neurological examination revealed no abnormal findings except mild left-sided limb weakness (MRC grade IV). Anti-phospholipid antibody and anti-SSA antibody were positive. Rheumatologist diagnosed her as antiphospholipid antibody syndrome. There were no significant findings in the transthoracic echocardiography, transesophageal echocardiography and Holter monitoring.

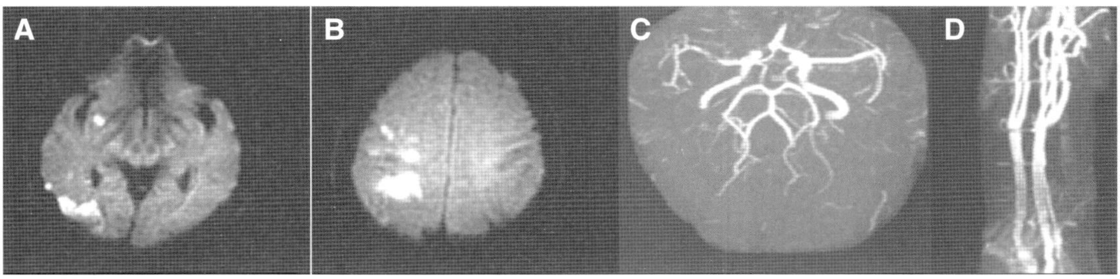

Brain MR-DWI (A, B) showed acute infarctions in the right MCA territory (insula, basal ganglia and temporoparietal lobe). Brain MRA (C, D) showed a focal stenosis of the right MCA stem and no stenosis in the neck vessels. She was treated with anticoagulant. Her weakness was not improved very much.

The stroke mechanism was thought to be an artery to artery embolism. Intracranial stenosis is a typical manifestation in antiphospholipid antibody syndrome. Antiphospholipid antibody is known to act in concert with other vascular risk factors, which damage endothelial cells and can cause cerebral ischemia.[24] But in this case, there was no risk factor of atherosclerosis. It is possible that anti-phospholipid antibody makes a direct contribution to the development of thrombosis.

• Case 112

A 60-year-old right-handed man came to our hospital for an abnormal speech. He had not any vascular risk factors, but had suffered nasopharyngeal cancer with lymph node metastasis receiving radical neck dissection and radiotherapy 20 years before. He had been in state of good health thereafter, but started to make an incoherent reply 8 days prior to admission. He spoke same phrase repetitively, and could not understand what others told. He had a sensory aphasia with impairment of naming and comprehension. There was a right homonymous hemianopsia, but no weakness or hypesthesia in the face and limbs. There were no abnormal findings in the transthoracic echocardiography and Holter monitoring. Transesophageal echocardiography was not done due to poor cooperation.

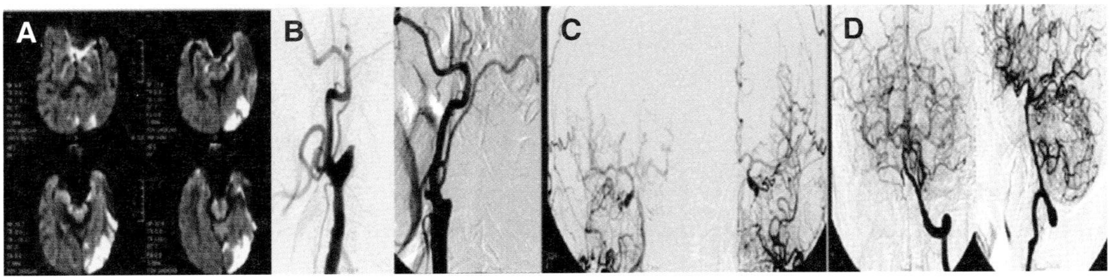

Brain MR-DWI (A) showed an acute infarction in the left temporo-occipital lobe and the right occipital lobe. Conventional angiography (B-D) showed complete bilateral occlusions of proximal ICA with collaterals through OA and Pcom. In addition, an anomalous tortuosity of the distal BA was noted. He took dual antiplatelet agents, aspirin and clopidogrel, and was discharged in state of right inferior quadrantanopsia and somewhat improved language function 1 month later.

The occlusion of bilateral proximal ICA was likely to be a complication of previous radiotherapy. Considering recanalized PCA flow on the angiography, this stroke mechanism was an embolization to PCA from unknown origin such as proximal VA, aortic arch and heart. Although it is not impossible for embolus to migrate through Pcom to MCA, sensory aphasia is through to originate from occlusion of PCA which gave collateral flow to the lateral temporal lobe since proximal ICA occlusion.

• Case 113

A 17-year-old right-handed man presented with a sudden onset of right arm weakness and dysarthria while attending a lecture. Weakness had persisted for 4 days and disappeared 1 day before admission. 1 month prior to the episode, he had experienced a sudden left visual field defect, which was slowly improved to complete recovery over 3 days. He had no significant past medical history. There was no abnormal finding in the neurologic examination except bilaterally equivocal Babinski signs and right carotid bruit. ECG, echocardiogram and Holter monitoring were all normal.

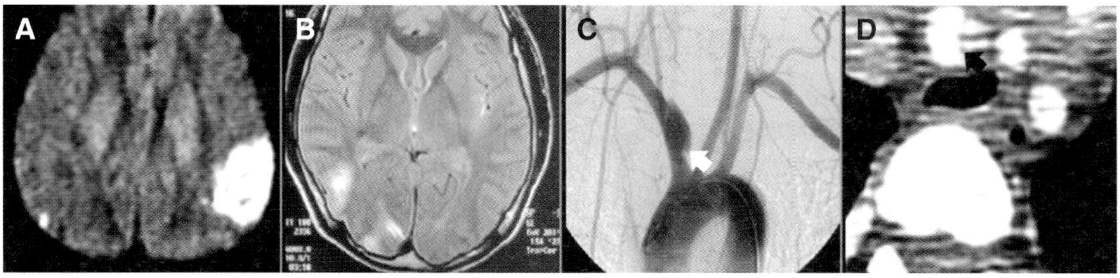

Brain MRI (A, B) showed acute infarctions in the bilateral posterior parietal lobe, mainly on the left. Conventional angiography (C) showed a complete occlusion in the right CCA and an aneurysmal dilatation in the right innominate artery (white arrow). CT angiography (D) revealed dissection of right innominate artery with CCA occlusion (black arrow). There was no subjective symptom initially. He was treated with an antiplatelet agent.

This patient had no stroke risk factor. The previous lesion of the right parietooccipital areas resulted from the right innominate artery dissection, with a possible distal embolizaton via Pcom. However, the left parietal lesion was thought to be an embolic infarction from unknown origin. We can see the intimal flap in TFCA and the true and false lumen in CT angiography.

• Case 114

A 48-year-old man complained of severe headache. He was a current smoker, and had a medical history of hypertension, which was well-controlled, but no history of head and neck trauma. 14 days prior to admission, he had felt a sudden pain on the posterior neck and the occiput in a moment of anger. It was sharp and continuous accompanied by nausea and vomiting. He had suffered a transient left hemiparesis for 10 minutes and eyeball deviation to the right side without loss of consciousness for a few minutes. Vital signs were within normal range. Neurologic examination revealed only a gaze-evoked nystagmus on the left gaze. There was no visual field defect, motor or sensory symptom in the face, dysarthria, or dysphagia. In laboratory tests, abnormal findings were not observed. ECG and echocardiography were normal.

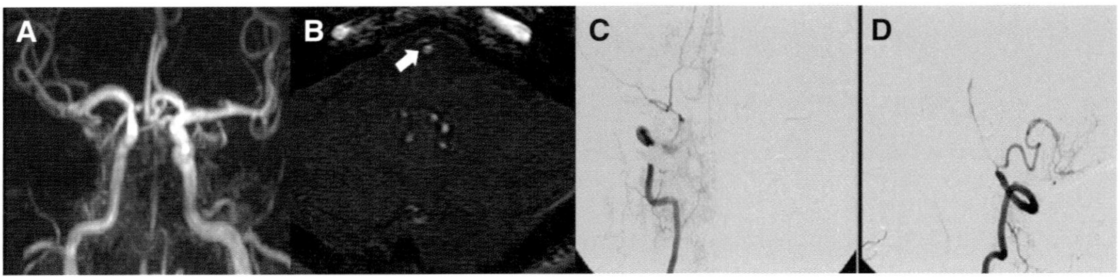

Initial brain MR-DWI did not have any abnormal finding. Brain MRA (A) identified a severe stenosis of the vertebro-BA. We could find a dissected left VA to be propagated through the vertebrobasilar junction to the left VA in TOF source image (B), which was also proven in conventional angiography (C, D). Because his symptom was trivial, we managed him with an antiplatelet agent. However, he complained of a sudden dysarthria, limb weakness (MRC grade intravenous) and hypesthesia in the right side, and emotional liability. DWI revealed acute infarctions in the right pons and medulla, and GRE had thrombus in the left distal VA and basilar artery in the followed MRI. Immediate anticoagulation and stent insertion in the left VA were applied. He did not any other symptom afterwards, and was discharged in an improved state.

This case was thought to be a spontaneous dissection from the left distal VA to BA and subsequent thrombosis, which occluded perforator vessels of the vertebrobasilar arteries.

• Case 115

A 45-year-old man was admitted presenting with a sudden right-sided weakness and dysarthria. 1 week before admission, whirling type dizziness, and headache had occurred suddenly. After 3 days, he had recognized a right-sided weakness and dysarthria in the morning. His neurologic symptoms were fluctuating. He had no stroke risk factors except ex-smoker. Mental state was normal and cranial examination showed dysarthria without facial palsy. His motor power was MRC grade IV in the right side. Sensory examination and cerebellar function test were normal. Echocardiography was normal with ejection fraction 69%.

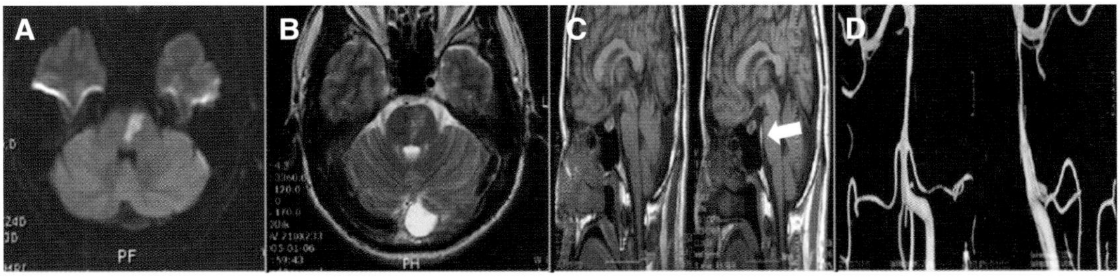

Brain MR-DWI (A) showed an acute infarction in the left paramedian pons. MRI (B, C) showed an effacement of vascular signal void, and intravascular hematoma (arrow), suggesting BA dissection. Conventional angiography (D) confirmed a dissection with irregular wall dilatation in the BA. He was given aspirin and later we added clopidogrel. His right-sided weakness improved.

The stroke mechanism was thought to be in situ thrombosis at the stenotic lesion of BA. The stenosis of BA was due to a spontaneous dissection.

• Case 116

A 30-year-old man presented with sudden dysarthria and gait disturbance after falling from a motorcycle 5 hours ago. He had no other medical diseases. The mental status was alert. In the cerebellar function test, he showed a limb ataxia on the right side and could not walk by himself. Cranial nerve examination and motor and sensory examination was normal. In laboratory tests, abnormal findings were not observed. ECG and echocardiography were normal.

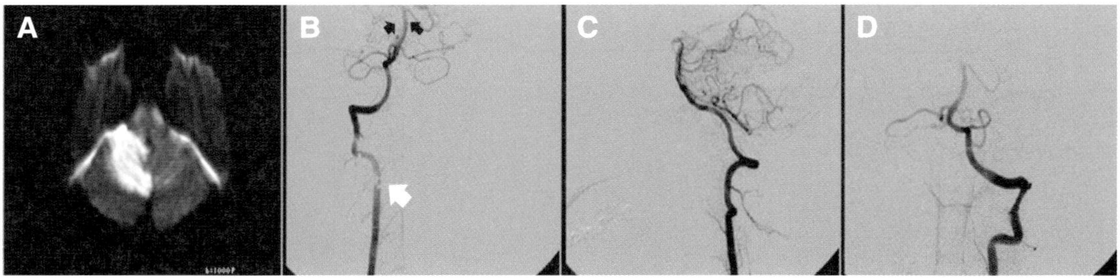

Brain MR-DWI (A) showed an acute infarct in the right SCA territory. In the conventional angiography (B-D), both SCA were not visualized (black arrows). Irregularity of the right distal VA with small pseudoaneurysm was also noted (white arrow). Left VA was intact, but distal flow disappeared at the distal level. Anticoagulation treatment was given to him, and any further attack did not recur thereafter.

The stroke mechanism was an artery to artery embolism resulting from the right VA dissection to the right SCA.

• Case 117

A 42-year-old woman presented with a sudden visual disturbance. 1 month before, during mountain climbing, she had suddenly felt visual disturbance in the left temporal side, followed by severe headache for subsequent 2 to 3 days. She had a history of migraine without aura but no definite risk factors for stroke. On the neurologic examination, the visual field defect was suspected on the left inferior temporal area. Motor, sensory, and language functions were intact. Transesophageal echocardiography showed a right to left shunt of microbubbles irrespective of valsalva maneuver and the microbubbles were drained to right pulmonary vein. During the valsalva maneuver, the microbubbles appeared in the left atrium with a delay of several cardiac cycles suggesting pulmonary arterio-venous fistula rather than PFO.

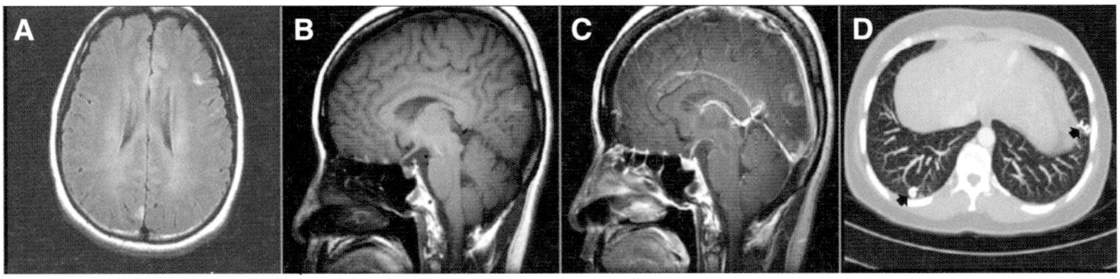

The FLAIR image (A) showed high signal intensities in the left frontal subcortical area and right striate cortex. These lesions were well-enhanced on T1WI (B, C). Chest CT (D) revealed multifocal pulmonary arteriovenous malformations (arrows). Brain MRA was normal. Transcranial Doppler showed multiple microemblic signals on agitated saline injection (latency: 10-15 sec.). Coil embolization was done for four arteriovenous malformations in both lungs.

The mechanism of stroke was thought to be a paradoxical embolism through right to left shunt caused by multiple pulmonary arteriovenous fistulas. The association of pulmonary arteriovenous fistula with stroke is known as Osler-Weber-Rendu disease, but exceptionally can be linked to pulmonary arteriovenous fistula without an O-W-R disease.[25]

• Case 118

A 59-year-old right-handed man presented with a sudden right-sided weakness and aphasia 1 day ago. He had a diabetes mellitus with insulin medication. And he had bladder cancer with multiple liver and bone metastasis. The language function test showed sensory dominant aphasia. Cranial nerve examination showed no remarkable findings. Motor power was MRC grade IV+. The sensory examination revealed a right-sided hypesthesia. Transthoracic echocardiography showed a septal asymmetrical hypertrophy without dynamic obstruction. Coagulation battery showed elevated FDP (1:5), D-dimer (2.45) (ref. < 0.4), and fibrinogen 601mg/dL.

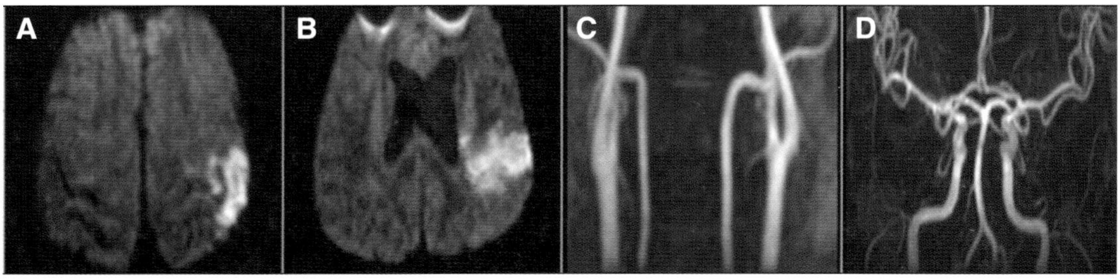

Brain MR-DWI (A, B) showed acute infarctions in the left MCA territory. Brain MRA (C, D) showed no significant stenoocclusive lesions. Aspirin was administered to this patient. Her symptoms were slowly improved.

He had known diabetes mellitus and metastatic bladder cancer. No embolic sources from the proximal carotid system or heart were detected. FDP and D-dimer levels were increased. The infarction in this patient was likely to result from underlying cancer-related hypercoagulable state.

• Case 119

A 61-year-old man was consulted from the department of thoracic surgery because of a left-sided weakness and altered mentality. 1 day before, he had undergone coronary artery bypass graft (CABG) surgery due to 2-vessel-disease. The next day his neurologic abnormalities were found. Neurologic examination revealed drowsy mental status, eyeball deviation to the right, left central-type facial palsy and left limb weakness (MRC grade I). Deep tendon reflex was hyperactive at the left side. Babinski sign was positive at the left side. Transthoracic echocardiography and Holter monitoring did not reveal any cardiac source of embolism.

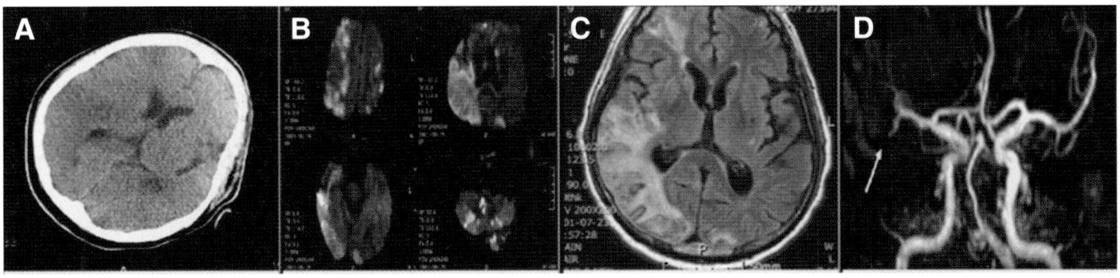

Brain CT (A) showed the obliteration of the right sulci. Brain MR-DWI (B) showed multiple acute infarctions in the right MCA, both PCA, both SCA and PICA territories, and left caudate nucleus. In the follow-up MRI and MRA, we could see the same lesion in the brain parenchyma (C) and an occlusion of the right MCA at the bifurcation (D). He was treated with antiplatelet agent and volume expansion. But, he has been in a bed-ridden state.

Stroke is a devastating complication of coronary artery bypass graft (CABG) surgery, with a reported incidence ranging from 1.3% to 4.3%.[26] Cardioembolism accounts for the majority of CABG-related strokes.

• Case 120

A 63-year-old man visited our hospital complaining of headache. He had had a head trauma in the middle of drinking alcohol 7 days before. Thereafter, he had suffered from a headache in the right hemicranial area. The nature of headache was pulsating, severe and continuous. 4 days before, he had felt a left-sided weakness. In the emergency room, he showed generalized tonic seizures for 1 minute. He had no previous medical history except head trauma. He showed a drowsy mentality and disorientation. Light reflex was normal and gaze preponderance to the right side was observed. In the motor system examination, right-sided weakness was MRC grade IV and left-sided was grade I. Deep tendon reflex was hyperreflexic in his left side. Neck-stiffness was not observed. In blood laboratory tests, there were no abnormalities in PT, Aptt, antithrombin III, protein C, protein S, plasminogen, lupus anticoagulant, and anti-phospholipid antibodies.

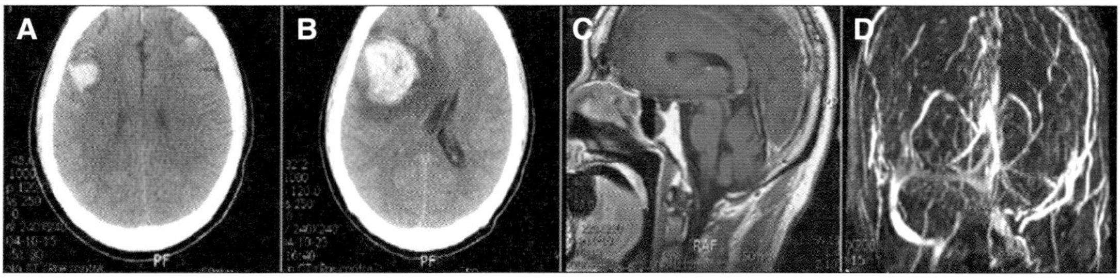

Brain CT (A, B) showed an acute hemorrhage with gyral swelling in both frontal lobes. T1WI (C) showed a massive thrombosis in the superior sagittal sinus with prominent cortical veins. In MR venography (D), massive thrombosis in superior sagittal sinus, left transverse, left sigmoid and right sphenoparietal vein with prominent cortical veins were observed. Anticoagulation with intravenous heparin and valporic acid medication was started. Brain CT was checked regularly and size of multiple intracerebral hemorrhages increased especially in right frontal lobe and we stopped anticoagulation because of mid-line shifting mass effect. After absorption of intracerebral hemorrhage volumes, he started rehabilitation and transferred to rehabilitation ward.

He had a prior trauma history and initial neurological symptom was headache. Minor head trauma can be a risk factor of cerebral venous thrombosis. Anticoagulation in the cerebral venous thrombosis with acute intracerebral hemorrhage may be controversial.

• Case 121

A 66-year-old man presented with an altered mental status. He had suffered from granulomatous vasculitis and received immunosuppressive treatment for 2 years. He had maintained medication of oral prednisolone 20mg twice a day. 2 days prior to admission, he had been disoriented with a visual hallucination, and then he progressively went into deep sleeping state. He was stuporous and showed a slight withdrawal response to pain. Light reflex, corneal reflex and vestibuloocular reflex were intact. Transthoracic echocardiography and Holter monitoring did not reveal any cardiac source of embolism.

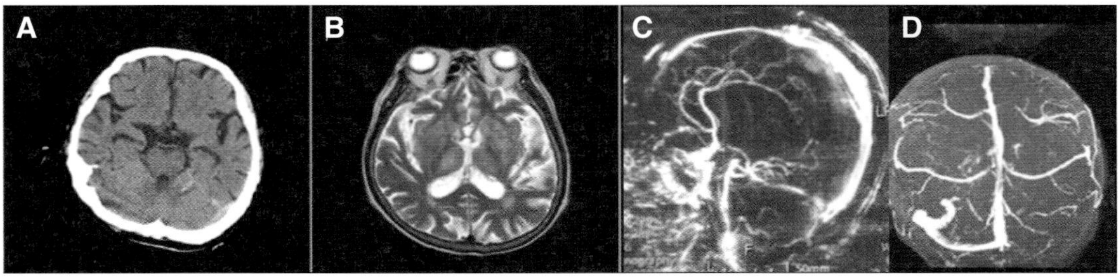

Brain CT (A) revealed a small amount of hemorrhagic density along sulci in the left cerebellum and increased attenuation in the left transverse sinus. Edematous swelling of deep gray matter was also seen. Acute T2 changes without definite DWI/ADC change in bilateral thalamus and basal ganglia were demonstrated on T2WI (B). MR venography (C, D) showed non-visualization of the left transverse sinus and straight sinus. He was treated with anticoagulant.

Cerebral venous thrombosis may complicate systemic inflammatory vasculitic disease as this case. Bilateral involvement of the thalamus, basal ganglia and surrounding white-matter suggests deep venous thrombosis. These lesions cause altered level of consciousness, bilateral long tract signs and sometimes decorticate or decerebrate posturing. Anticoagulants are not expected to influence an already formed thrombus, but they should at least theoretically prevent extension of thrombosis in other venous channels. Two randomized placebo-controlled studies have shown that it gives clinical improvement even in patients with hemorrhagic infarct, provided there are no contraindications.[27]

• Case 122

A 59-year-old man developed facial palsy and dysarthria suddenly 6 days before admission. He had been medicated with anti-hypertensive drug since 5 years ago. He had been diagnosed as thrombotic thrombocytopenic purpura. Past medical history included a left MCA infarction presenting with motor aphasia 1 year ago. He showed a left central-type facial palsy and dysarthria. His platelet count was 89,000/uL. Echocardiography showed no abnormalities.

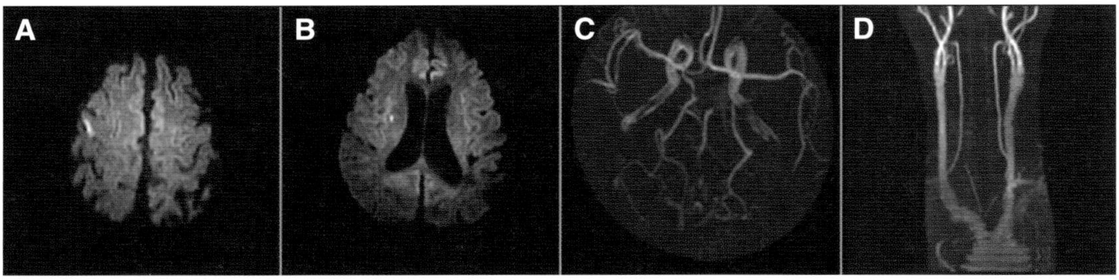

Brain MR-DWI (A, B) showed high signal intensities in the right precentral gyrus and corona radiate and prominent left temporoparietal gyri maybe due to old infarction. Brain MRA (C, D) showed no significant stenoocclusive lesions. His neurological symptom was nearly recovered. Initially, clopidogrel was started and low-dose warfarin was added.

He did not have any other stroke risk factor and we thought that the presumed stroke mechanism was thrombotic thrombocytopenic purpura.

• Case 123

A 51-year-old, right-handed woman presented with a sudden onset of dysarthria and right-sided weakness, which was developed 8 hours prior to visit. He had been diagnosed with Takayasu's arteritis and under medication of steroid and azathioprine for 8 years. She had no other risk factor of stroke. Her language function was normal. Speech was dysarthric. Mild weakness (MRC grade IV) involving the right limb and face was detected. Carotid bruit was audible bilaterally. Transthoracic echocardiography showed basal inferoseptal akinesia. Level of total cholesterol was 245mg/dL and ESR was mildly elevated to 24mm/hr.

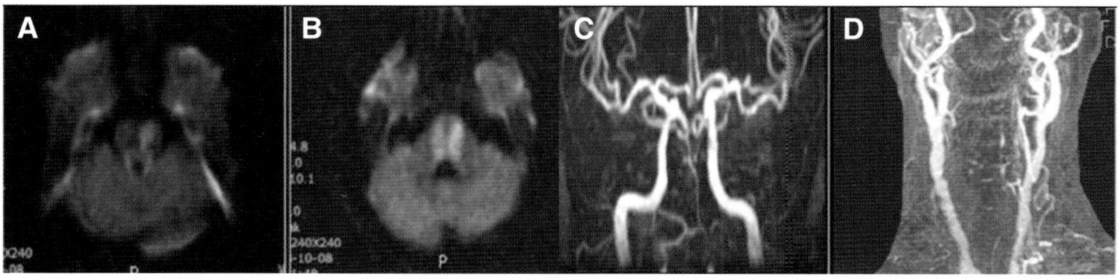

Brain MR-DWI (A, B) showed an acute infarction in the left pons. Brain MRA (C, D) showed a poor flow of both proximal VAs and both subclavian arteries. She was treated with dual antiplatelet agents, a lipid-lowering agent and steroid. Weakness and dysarthria was slightly improved.

The subclavian artery proximal to the origin of the VA is often involved earlier in the Takayasu's arteritis. The mechanism of stroke was thought to be an artery-to-artery embolism from the proximal VA or low flow phenomenon of the brainstem.

• Case 124

A 40-year-old woman was hospitalized due to intermittent headache, which had started 10 years prior to admission. The headache had a pulsating nature involving bilateral frontoparietal areas, lasting for about 3 hours. It was frequently accompanied with nausea. There was no definite aura. Her mother also had a history of similar headache. She had no stroke risk factors. There were no abnormal findings in the neurologic examination. Genetic test for the diagnosis of CADASIL was positive. The work-up for other causes of white matter disease yielded no significance. Gene test for family members of the patient was not performed. Transthoracic echocardiography and Holter monitoring did not reveal any cardiac source of embolism.

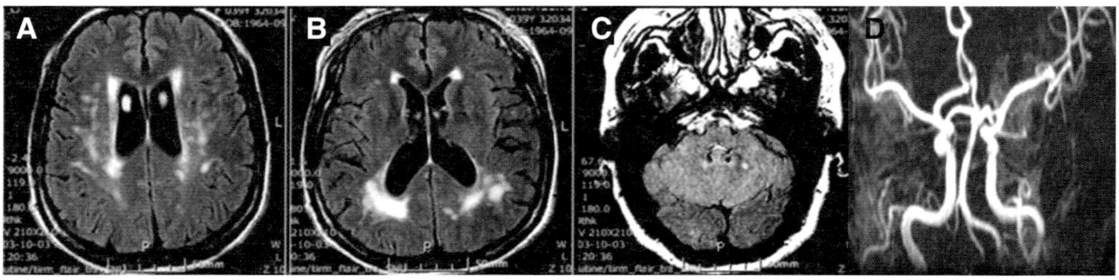

Brain MRI (A-C) showed multiple high signal intensities in the bilateral periventricular white matter and left cerebellum. Brain MRA (D) showed no significant stenosis in the intracranial and extracranial arteries. She was treated with amitriptyline and aspirin. There was a mild improvement of headache.

MRI showed nodular T2-high signal lesions with symmetrical distribution and the lesions predominated in the periventricular areas and centrum semiovale. Microbleeds were also frequently observed. Genetic study was compatible with CADASIL although the autosomal dominance was not confirmed. Migraine with aura is the earliest manifestation of CADASIL with a mean onset age of 28 years.[28]

• Case 125

A 52-year-old man presented with a sudden onset of right-sided weakness. 3 years prior to visit, he had experienced a sudden dysarthria and had been diagnosed with lacunar infarction. Right-sided weakness had developed abruptly 1 day before admission and aggravated progressively. He had no risk factors for stroke. History of migraine or mood disorder cannot be checked. Gene study confirmed CADASIL although skin biopsy was not compatible with CADASIL. Transthoracic echocardiography and Holter monitoring did not reveal any cardiac source of embolism.

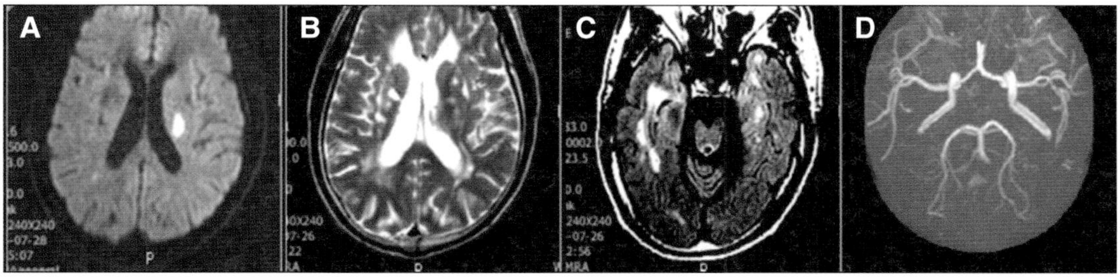

Brain MR-DWI (A) showed a small acute infarction in the left corona radiata. On MRI (B, C), old lesions were also demonstrated in periventricular white matter and basal ganglia, temporal lobe, and external capsule. Brain MRA (D) showed no significant stenoocclusive lesions. He was treated with an antiplatelet agent. Dysarthria and right-sided weakness was slightly improved.

Although he had no risk factors for atherosclerosis, there were multiple high signal intensity lesions in both periventricular white matter and basal ganglia on the T2WI. Lesions involving external capsule and anterior temporal lobe are seen frequently in CADASIL.[29] CADASIL can be considered as a diagnosis even though familial history was not definite and skin biopsy was not compatible.

• Case 126

A 27-year-old woman was admitted to our hospital presenting with right leg jerky movement. Right leg jerky movement had developed suddenly 2 days before. She had a history of developmental delay and mental retardation. She had suffered from a slowly progressive dysarthria and gait disturbance for 8-9 years. Seizure had developed 5 years before. Visual hallucination had developed 4 years before. She had been admitted to neurology ward 2 times due to intractable seizures. Mental status, cranial nerves, sensory system, and cerebellar function exams were normal. Motor power was MRC grade IV in four extremities. Muscle biopsy revealed denervation atrophy. CSF lactic acid was measured 5.2mmol/L. Gene test for MELAS was positive.

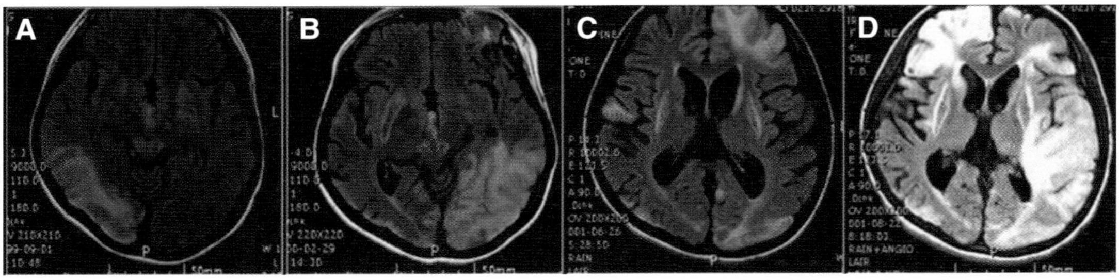

Right temporo-occipital and left fronto-temporal-occipital T2 high signal intensity lesions were aggravated on serial brain MRI (A-D). Her right leg jerky movement disappeared with valproic acid and carbamazepine. In the EEG, this symptom was related to a small amount of ictal discharges in both temporal lobes.

MELAS includes lactic acidosis and stroke-like episodes. Lactic acid is more sensitive in CSF. In MRS, increased lactate peak in the lateral ventricle is observed in patients with MELAS. Pathophysiology of stroke-like lesions in a patient with MELAS is controversial; cytotoxic edema or vasogenic edema.[30]

• Case 127

A 30-year-old man was admitted presenting with aphasia. 5 days before admission, he had had difficulty in understanding words. This symptom had developed suddenly. There were no motor weakness, sensory change and dysarthria. In past medical history, he had experienced a sudden left-sided weakness, tingling, and dysarthria. Also, he had suffered generalized tonic clonic seizures several times. He had a hearing loss from early childhood. However, he had no history of diabetes mellitus, hypertension, and smoking. His consciousness was alert and orientation was intact. Aphasia was absent. In cranial nerve examination, he showed sensorineural hearing loss bilaterally. Motor system and reflex system were normal. He revealed mild hypesthesia in his left arm. Arterial lactate concentration was 4.1mmol/L (0.7-2.5mmol/L) and CSF lactate concentration was 4.2mmol/L. Muscle biopsy revealed ragged red fibers consistent with mitochondrial myopathy. Gene test was positive.

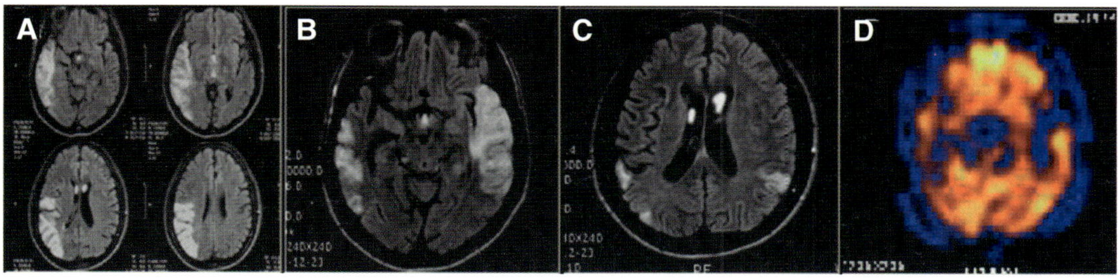

MRI (A-C) showed high signal intensity changes in both parieto-temporo-occipital lobes over 2 years. Brain MRA showed no significant stenoocclusive lesions. Brain SPECT (D) revealed decreased perfusion in both temporal lobes. He was given evaporate and aspirin.

MELAS is a mitochondrial encephalopathy with lactic acidosis and stroke-like episodes. In young patients with ischemic stroke, MELAS must be considered. This patient showed lesions not compatible with arterial territories and the lesion size was decreased with minimal cerebromalacia. Brain SPECT showed hyperperfusion until 4 weeks after disease onset and 4 weeks later showed hypoperfusion.

• Case 128

A 20-year-old man visited our hospital due to seizure. 10 days before, he had had a sudden thunderclap headache at the left occipital area with nausea and vomiting. The headache had repeatedly occurred several times with duration of 2-3 minutes. 3 days before, he had suddenly lost his consciousness for 20 seconds, accompanied by eyeball deviation rightward. There was neither aura nor convulsive movement. He had complained of bilateral visual disturbance and hearing difficulty since several years ago. He had had an end stage renal disease on hemodialysis since 1 year ago. At the time of admission, he was alert but had acalculia, finger agnosia and right-left disorientation (Gertsmann feature). He also had right homonymous hemianopsia and mild dysarthria. Motor and sensory examinations were normal. Deep tendon reflexes were hyperactive bilaterally. EEG showed no abnormality. Lactic acid levels were elevated in the serum and CSF. Through the genetic study, mitochondrial DNA mutation of 3243 was found.

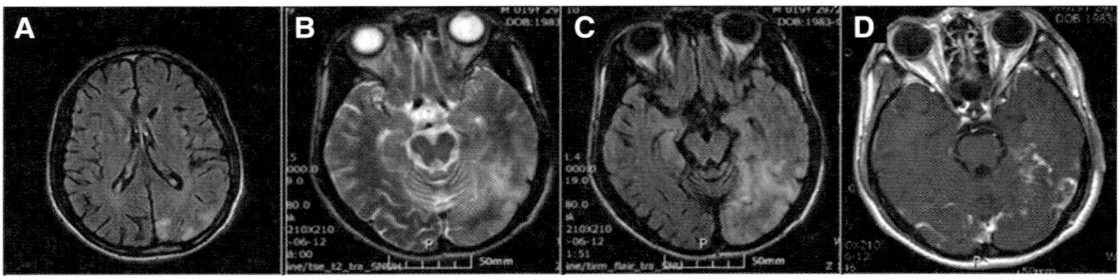

Primary MRI (A) showed a subacute infarction in the left parietal temporal area. 1 year later, the lesion was extended to both temporal lobes (B-D). Brain MRA was within normal limit. He was diagnosed as MELAS. He was given conservative management.

Focal lesions in MELAS patients are mostly in the parieto-occipital lobes mainly involving cortex and not confined to the vascular territory. Stroke or stroke-like episodes are the most striking feature but, episodic vomiting, sudden episode of headache and seizures are common in MELAS syndrome. The mechanisms leading to stroke episodes in MELAS are not known at present.

• Case 129

A 59-year-old woman presented with a sudden pain around neck and left posterior auricular area, followed by a dull-natured headache. The MR angiogram performed in other hospital revealed abnormal findings. She was referred to our hospital. Her past medical history included no risk factors for stroke. Neurological examination showed no abnormality except carotid bruit on the left side. In laboratory tests, abnormal findings were not observed. ECG and echocardiography were normal.

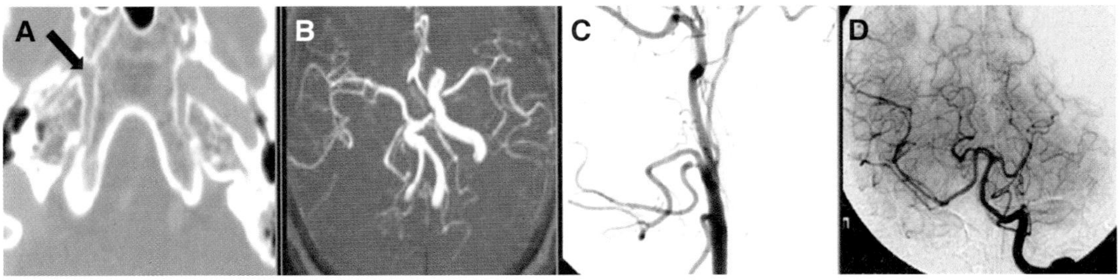

Temporal bone CT (A) showed an absence of the right carotid canal (arrow). Brain MRA (B) and conventional angiography (C, D) showed an absence of the right ICA. The right ACA and MCA were supplied from contralateral ICA and posterior circulation via Pcom, respectively. The angiographic findings were incidental and not related to her symptoms. She was taken care with symptomatic treatment. Her symptoms improved and she was discharged.

Agenesis, aplasia, and hypoplasia of the ICA are rare congenital anomalies, occurring in less than 0.01% of the population.[31] The pattern of collateral blood flow to the distal ICA and intracranial vasculature is dependent upon the stage at which the disruption occurred. Demonstrating an absent or diminutive carotid canal with skull base CT will permit one to differentiate the congenital ICA anomaly from acquired condition resulting in a small-caliber ICA. The reported prevalence of the aneurysm in association with absence of the ICA is 24% to 34%.[31] Increased flow through collateral vessels and altered flow dynamics are cited as plausible explanation. Acom is the most frequent site of aneurysm formation in such cases.

• Case 130

A 64-year-old man was admitted to our hospital due to a sudden right-sided weakness. 18 years before admission, he had experienced a left hemiparesis. In addition, he had had an acute myocardial infarction 10 years before. He had been on anticoagulation since 4 years prior to admission. 1 year before, he had developed post-stroke seizure and had been on antiepileptic medication. He showed a right central-type facial palsy and right facial hypesthesia. Motor and sensory examination revealed a right-sided weakness (MRC grade IV) and hypesthesia. Laboratory finding showed no abnormal findings but elevated high homocysteine level (62mg/dL).

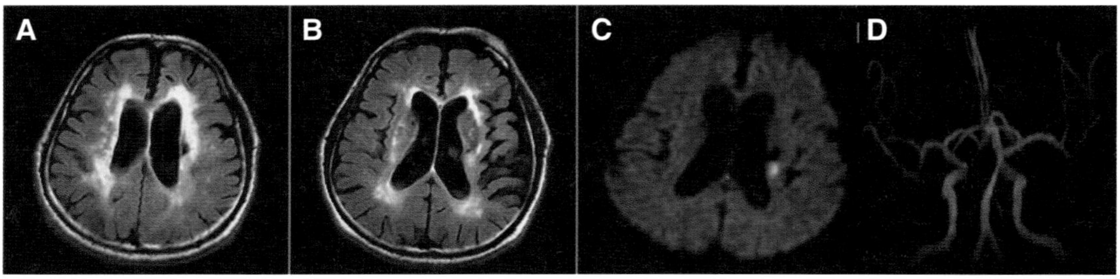

Brain MR-FLAIR images (A, B) showed multiple lacunes with leukoaraiosis. On DWI (C), new lacunar stroke was demonstrated in the left corona radiata. Brain MRA (D) showed no vascular abnormalities. He was treated with folate and cyanocobalamin. His homocysteine level was normalized.

He had no vascular risk factors. His homocysteine level was high. In this patient, high level of homocysteine was a cause of ischemic lesion. Elevated homocysteine is associated with a higher risk of cerebrovascular disease.[32] However, it remains controversial whether lowering of homocysteine with folic acid and vitamins B6 and B12 reduces the risk of stroke, stroke severity or disability.

• Case 131

A 31-year-old woman presented with an impaired level of consciousness. She had been in a good health through her whole life, and was 34-week pregnant. Recently, she had suffered generalized edema, and proteinuria. She had not shown any abnormal features until that morning, but was found comatose by her husband in the evening. She had a generalized tonic-clonic seizure and cardiac arrest, and was resuscitated with giving a stillbirth at local hospital. She showed limb flexion to pain stimuli, but did not open eye. Cranial nerve examination was normal including light reflex and doll's eye. There was bilaterally brisk deep tendon reflex and positive toe sign. EEG revealed arrhythmic delta slowing in all leads without spike.

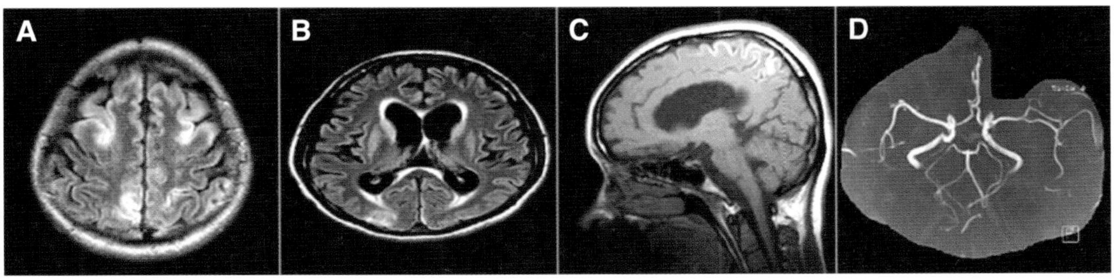

MRI (A, B) showed high signal lesions in both frontal and parietooccipital areas with increased cortical enhancement (C), suggesting BBB breakdown. Brain MRA (D) showed no stenosis in the intracranial vessels. She became alert, but did not respond to outer stimuli. Generalized edema and proteinuria slowly improved, and her BP was well-controlled after stillbirth. No more seizure was observed. A follow-up MRI after 2 weeks revealed a slight resolution of the previous lesions with some high signals in subcortical area.

We could infer from the high ADC that the high signal of MRI was due to vasogenic edema. This case was a hypertensive encephalopathy (one of the causes of Posterior Reversible Encephalopathy Syndrome; PRES), which occurred as a result of eclampsia. A significant fall in cerebrovascular resistance and a loss of autoregulation resulting in cerebral overperfusion was thought to be the mechanism.

IV

Interesting and Instructive Cases

• Case 132

A 67-year-old right-handed man presented for a sudden right-sided weakness. He had a medical history of atrial fibrillation, and had taken aspirin, digoxin and furosemide. On that day, in the middle of gambling, he suddenly showed the right limb weakness and did not respond to any question. He was admitted to local hospital being treated with intravenous rt-PA and transferred to our emergency room. He was drowsy and in global aphasic state. The neurologic examination revealed right side facial palsy, hemiplegia, and gaze preponderance to the left. Atrial fibrillation was noted on ECG. Echocardiography showed a left atrium dilation without definite thrombus.

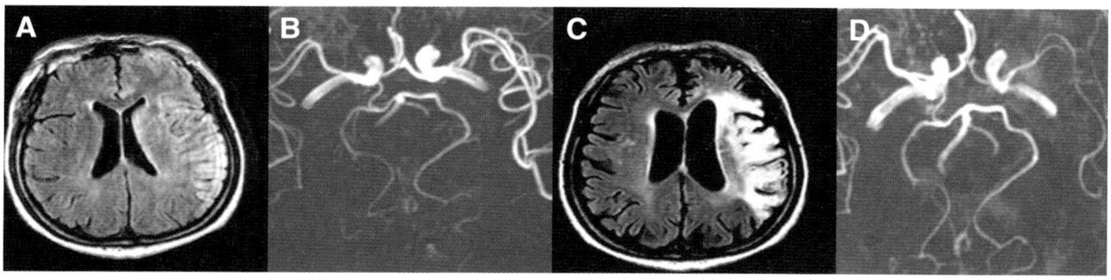

MRI (A) showed an acute infarction in the left MCA territory. Brain MRA (B) did not show any severe stenotic area in the MCA, but slightly increased flow signal of the MCA compared to the right side, maybe due to post-ischemic hyperperfusion. In the follow up MRI/A after 3 months (C, D), we could see a decreased flow signal on the left MCA and old left MCA infarction, which spared the lenticulostriate artery territory. He was treated with warfarin, and did not show any recurrent stroke event. His motor power improved to MRC grade IV. He was able to understand one or two phrase, but couldn't speak any word until discharge.

The initial brain MRA showed so-called "luxury perfusion; postischemic hyperperfusion" which means the early angiographic blush of recanalized brain infarction characterized by increased CBV and decreased oxygen extraction in excess of demand.[33] But, the decreased flow signal in the follow-up brain MRA indicates a reduction of metabolic demand in the MCA territory.

• Case 133

An 83-year-old woman was referred to department of neurology for a sudden left-sided weakness. She had experienced recurrent transient left-sided weakness three and 2 months prior to admission, and had been managed with clopidogrel, atorvastatin, and irbesartan. However, she had been operated on breast ductal carcinoma in spite of our recommendation of management for the severe proximal ICA stenosis, which was detected on preoperative brain MRA. On the second day after operation, she was detected to be in state of loss of consciousness and to have a left limb weakness in the middle of defecation. Her systolic BP was 70mmHg and heart rate was 60/min at that time, but they were stabilized soon after. She was slightly drowsy with intact orientation, and had facial palsy, motor weakness (MRC grade II), hypesthesia and visual field defect in the left side. She also showed asomatognosia for the left limb and gaze preponderance to the right side. ECG and echocardiography were all normal and carotid bruit was noted on the right side.

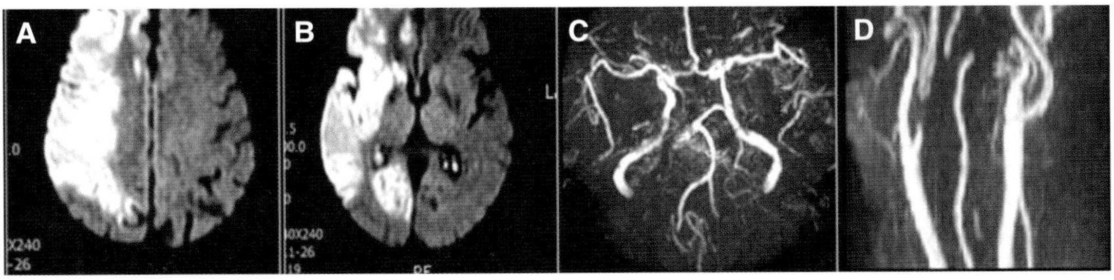

Brain MR-DWI (A, B) showed an acute infarction in the right MCA and PCA territories. Brain MRA (C, D) showed a severe stenosis in the right proximal ICA, severe stenosis in the right PCA with fetal circulation, and segmental stenosis in right distal ICA. She had a persistent limb weakness in spite of intravenous rt-PA. On the next day, she showed decreased mentality and dilated right side pupil. Subsequent brain CT revealed an increased brain edema with midline shift. She underwent decompression surgery with mannitol and pentothal coma therapy.

The stroke mechanism was an artery to artery embolism from the proximal ICA. Large and panhemispheric infarctions generally result from embolic infarction. Hypotension and postoperative dehydration is likely to induce low flow stroke under hemodynamic compromise or thrombus propagation in the unstable plaque.

• Case 134

A 64-year-old woman was admitted because of a sudden dysarthria and decreased verbal response. She also complained of a left hand weakness. 3 years before admission, she had suffered from hypertension and diabetes mellitus with irregular medication. She had no history of heart disease or previous stroke. She was alert and oriented but with apathy and abulia. There was no motor or visual neglect on the left side. Cranial nerve examinations were normal except for mild dysarthria. His left upper extremity was weak (MRC grade IV-). Sensory examination showed no abnormal findings. Ataxia, tremor and gait abnormality were not noted. Transthoracic echocardiography and Holter monitoring did not reveal any cardiac source of embolism.

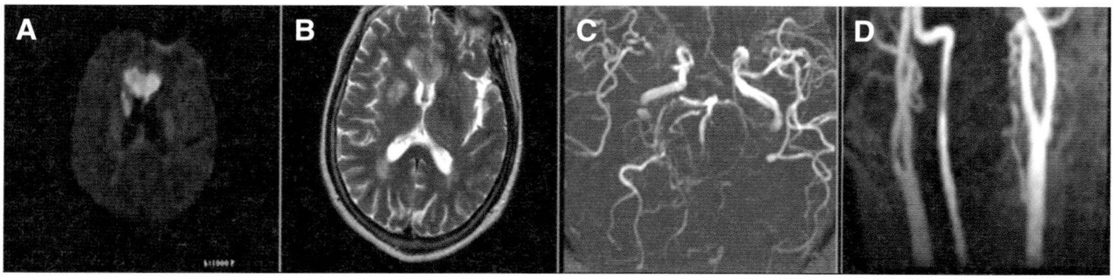

Brain MR-DWI (A, B) showed multiple infarcts involving right caudate and bilateral corpus callosum. Brain MRA (C, D) showed right A1 total occlusion, left A1 stenosis and right M1 severe stenosis. Hypertension and diabetes mellitus were well controlled. She was treated with dual antiplatelet agents.

Bilateral asymmetric ACA infarcts resulted from disease of the dominant right ACA. The caudate nucleus is supplied from right recurrent artery of Heubner or lenticulostriate artery of MCA. Therefore, the most plausible stroke mechanism was in situ thrombosis of the right ACA. However, an artery to artery embolism from the atheromatous proximal to the right ACA is also possible.

• Case 135

A 44-year-old man presented with a sudden right hemiparesis. The weakness had progressed over initial several hours. At the time of admission, he could not respond to environment and had a decreased verbal output. He also had urinary retention. He had a history of diabetes mellitus and hyercholesterolemia. He was alert, but showed abulia and akinesia. Orientation and verbal obey command was intact. He had a right central-type facial palsy and right hemiplegia. Sensory was also impaired for all modalities on the right side. ECG and echocardiography showed no abnormality.

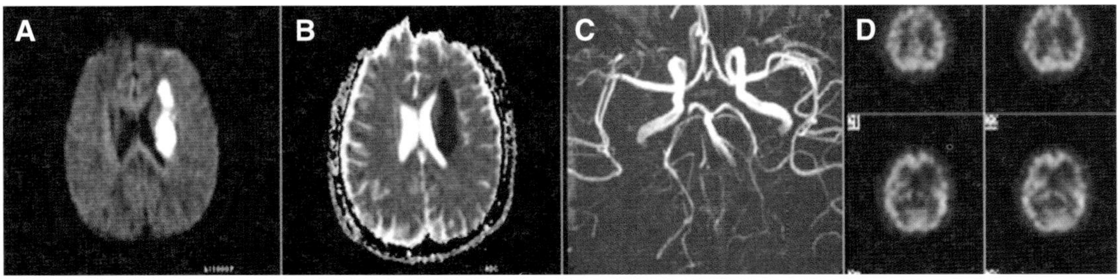

Brain MR-DWI and ADC (A, B) showed an acute infarction in the left periventricular white matter and basal ganglia. Brain MRA (C) revealed focal stenoses in the bilateral MCA. Brain SPECT (D) revealed decreased perfusion and vascular reserve in the white matter of left frontal lobe and left basal ganglia, which was much larger than infarcted area on MRI. He was treated with an antiplatelet agent. Frontal lobe dysfunction such as akinesia, abulia and neurogenic bladder persisted for more than 2 weeks.

The mechanism of stroke was thought to be embolism rather than in situ thrombosis. But embolic source was not found in spite of extensive work-ups. Neurological symptoms and signs can present beyond lesions on DWI. Occasionally, perfusion study would be better to delineate the dysfunctional regions.

• Case 136

A 64-year-old man visited our emergency room because of a sudden left-sided weakness. He had a history of hypertension and diabetes mellitus with regular medication, and had taken an antiplatelet agent. On the day of admission, he realized a left limb weakness on awakening, which was not changed until examination. He had a central-type facial palsy and limb weakness (MRC grade III/IV) in the left side. The ECG and echocardiography did not show any abnormal finding.

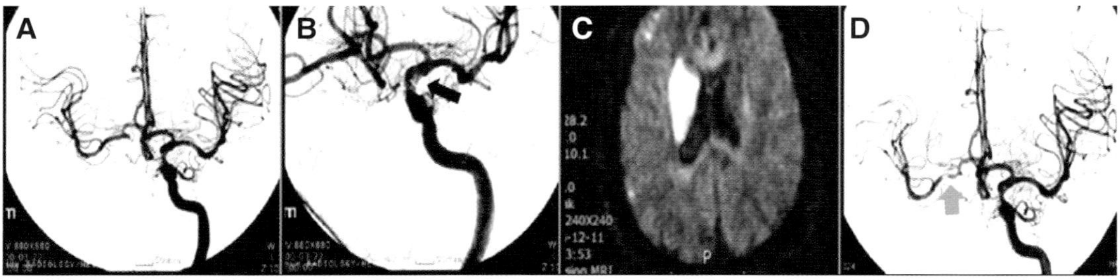

His previous angiography (A, B) before this attack showed a complete occlusion of right proximal ICA and unstable plaque of the left distal ICA (black arrow). Brain MR-DWI (C) showed an acute infarction in the right basal ganglia and cortex. At this admission, conventional angiography (D) demonstrated a thrombus in the right MCA stem (grey arrow). He was given aspirin and clopidogrel. The weakness did not much improve at discharge.

Considering a complete occlusion of the right proximal ICA and unstable plaque of left distal ICA, we think the presumed mechanism of stroke is an artery to artery embolization from the left distal ICA via Acom to the right MCA.

• Case 137

A 46-year-old man visited our hospital for a sudden left-sided weakness and tingling sensation. He had a previous medical history of 1-year hypertension. 7 days prior to admission, he had felt a left-sided weakness and tingling sensation with continuous vertigo after bathing. He had been treated at the local hospital, but the limb weakness had progressed. So he was referred to our hospital. Neurologic examination revealed a left-sided weakness (MRC grade IV) and hypesthesia. There was no definite nystagmus or limitation of the eye of movement. Deep tendon reflex was hyperactive and babinski sign was positive on the left. The ECG and echocardiography did not show any abnormal finding.

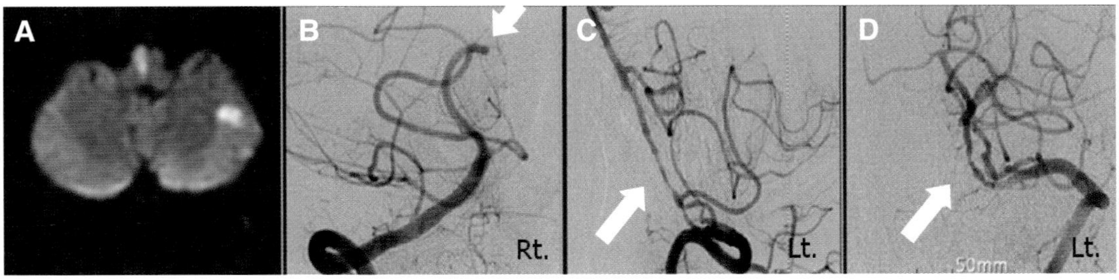

Brain MR-DWI (A) showed acute ischemic infarctions in the right side of the medulla oblongata and left cerebellar hemisphere. Conventional angiography (B-D) showed a termination of the right VA at the V-B junction and a severe stenosis on the left VA and BA (arrows). He was treated with an anticoagulant due to aggravation of the limb weakness.

The stroke mechanism of this patient was an artery to artery embolization which may be from the left VA to the PICA in the left cerebellum and to the anterior spinal artery in the right median medulla.

• Case 138

A 66-year-old woman presented with a sudden confused mentality. She had no motor or sensory symptom. She had taken anticoagulant since the last year because of atrial fibrillation combined with mitral valve regurgitation. She had a hypertension with congestive heart failure. She was alert, but sensory aphasia was observed. Cranial nerve functions and motor power were intact. PT-INR was 1.89.

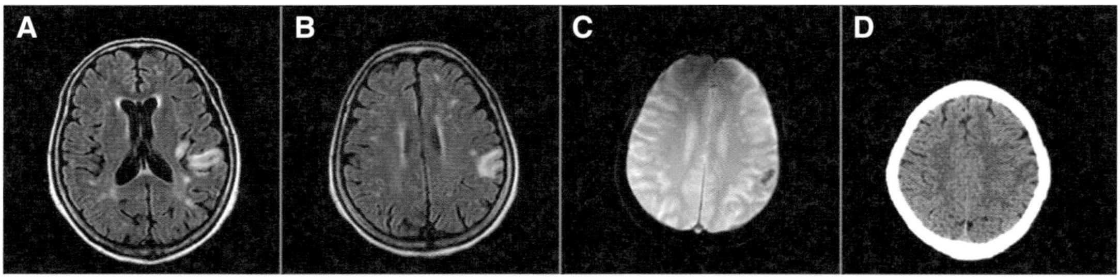

MRI (A-D) showed multiple acute infarctions with some hemorrhagic component in the left frontoparietal cortex and subcortical areas of the frontoparietal lobe and bilateral posterior insular area, compatible with embolic infarct. Brain MRA showed no significant stenoocclusive lesions. She had been on warfarin medication and warfarin dose adjustment was needed.

The mechanism of stroke was a cardioembolism. Atrial fibrillation accompanied by mitral regurgitation in congestive heart failure is a high risk for cardioembolism. Hemorrhagic infarction with no definite corresponding proximal vascular lesion strongly suggests embolic infarction. In spite of anticoagulation, this patient suffered multiple embolic infarctions. In this case, the INR should be adjusted to somewhat upper range.

• Case 139

A 63-year-old woman developed a sudden left-sided weakness 2 days before admission. She had a history of 20-year hypertension and transient ischemic attack 10 years ago. She had taken triflusal for 4 years. She felt a left-sided weakness and numbness during doing the housework. The symptom was stationary till admission. She showed a left central-type facial hypesthesia, dysarthria, left-sided weakness (MRC grade IV+) and left-sided hemibody hypesthesia. The toe sign of the left was extensor. The transthoracic echocardiography, transesophageal echocardiography and transcranial Doppler were all within normal limits.

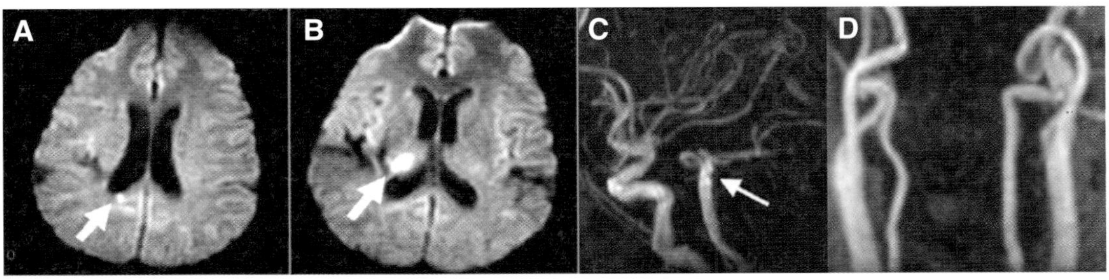

Brain MR-DWI (A, B) showed multiple infarctions in the right dorsolateral thalamus and splenium. Brain MRA (C) showed a focal irregular vascular change in the distal BA (arrow). Neck vessel (D) was intact. Aspirin was added to this patient and the symptom was improved steadily.

The most common etiology of the lateral thalamic territory infarction is a small vessel disease, and the embolic infarction of the thalamus usually is located in medial portion. However, this stroke mechanism of the patient was an artery to artery embolization from distal BA to PCA, because of a concomitant small infarction in the posterior corpus callosum (splenium).

• Case 140

A 69-year-old man presented with a sudden onset of dizziness and headache. He had not been able to walk because of dizziness 3 days prior to visit. About 19 years before, he had experienced abrupt visual disturbance to be diagnosed with right PCA infarction. He had suffered from diabetes mellitus, hyperlipidemia and hypertension for about 30 years. Aspirin was included in his medication. He was alert. Horner features were detected on the right side. The examination of extraocular movement showed left lateropulsion and mixed torsional nystagmus to the left side. Gaze-evoked nystagmus to the right side was also noted. Dysphagia, hoarseness and ataxia on the right side were evident. Left visual field defect and mild left-sided weakness (MRC grade IV+) were noted but thought to be sequelae of old stroke. Bruit was not audible. Transthoracic echocardiography was normal.

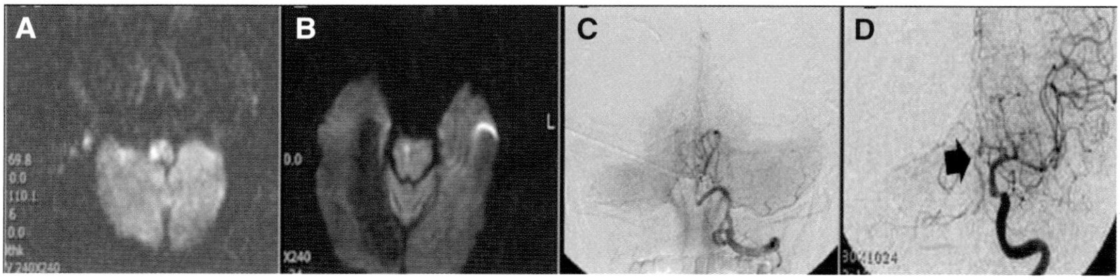

Brain MR-DWI (A, B) showed acute infarctions in the right lateral medulla. Heparinization was started but stopped due to gross hematuria. He was treated with clopidogrel and aspirin. About 1 month after admission, he complained of a left-sided weakness. Follow-up DWI (B) showed an acute pontine infarction. Conventional angiography (C, D) showed a complete occlusion of right VA, unclear termination of the left VA, and collateral posterior circulation from the left ICA to BA via Pcom (arrow). Anticoagulation was started again. Dysphagia and weakness was slightly improved when he was discharged.

There was no evidence of cardioembolism. Considering hypoplastic vertebrobasilar system with retrograde flow from left ICA, the mechanism of stroke was thought to be in situ thrombosis or low flow.

• Case 141

A 68-year-old woman was consulted to the department of neurology for altered mentality. 1 day before the consult, insidious drowsiness had been developed. She had been admitted in the department of internal medicine for known rectal cancer with lung and bone metastasis. Miles operation and palliative radiotherapy had been done. On examination, she was semicomatose, anisocoric (5mm/3mm), but doll's eye movements and facial grimacing to pain stimuli were symmetric and intact. Limb withdrawals to pain stimuli were symmetric above MRC grade III and deep tendon reflex revealed hyperactivity, but toe signs were flexor on both feet. Neck flexion was rigid. Transthoracic echocardiography and Holter monitoring did not reveal any cardiac source of embolism.

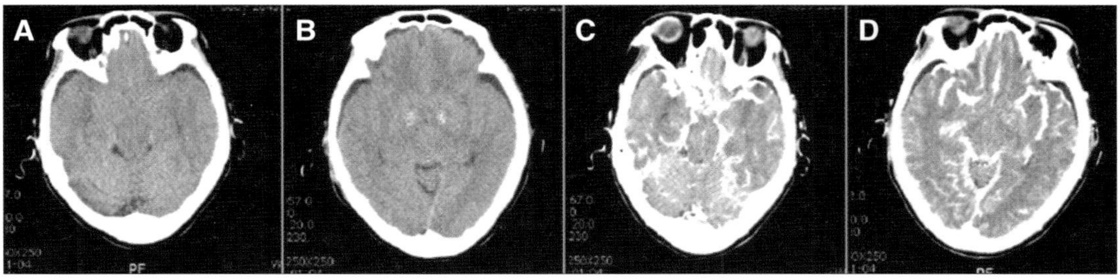

Brain CT (A-D) revealed progressive brain edema, basal cistern obliteration, and engorged venous enhancement. We thought the brainstem compression was the cause of altered mentality, so mannitol was used for controlling of intracranial pressure. Anticoagulation was also considered. But the next day, she expired with respiratory arrest.

We thought the cause of her drowsy mentality was a brainstem compression by cerebral edema due to thrombosis of deep cerebral veins.

• Case 142

A 55-year-old man came to emergency room for a sudden left-sided weakness. He was a 20-pack-year current smoker, and had a medical history of hypertension, which was not treated. 2 days before admission, he had developed sudden left limb weakness, numbness, and dysarthria in the middle of bus tour. However, he did not have any symptoms of headache, nausea and vomiting. The BP was 200/110mmHg on arrival, but other vital sign was within normal range. He showed limb weakness (MRC grade IV) and hypesthesia on the left side. We could not detect any other abnormal finding on routine laboratory, coagulation test, and cardiac work-ups.

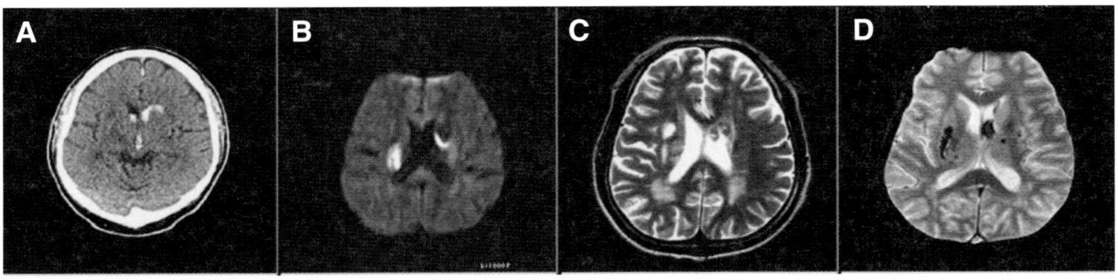

There were an acute infarction in the right corona radiata and acute intracerebral hemorrhage in the left caudate nucleus with intraventricular hemorrhage (A, B). The T2WI (C) and GRE image (D) revealed a lot of lacunes and microbleeds in both basal ganglia. Brain MRA did not show any vascular abnormality. We had a difficulty in keeping the BP in control in spite of antihypertensive drugs.

The symptom of left-sided weakness resulted from an acute lacunar infarction in the right corona radiata. In addition, we could find a coincidental acute hemorrhage in the left caudate nucleus extending into the third ventricle. Considering the iso or slightly low signal in T2-weighted MR image, the hemorrhage was thought to be in acute stage which occurred at the same time as the lacune. This situation combined with infarction and hemorrhage requires more careful attention to treatment.

• Case 143

A 67-year-old man was admitted to the emergency department because of a sudden visual disturbance while watching a television. He noticed that the inferior half of the right eye field was defected. He had a history of hypertension, hypercholesterolemia, and heavy smoking of 40 packyears. Neurologic examination revealed a visual field defect on the inferior half of the right eye. Visual perception of the left eye was normal. Other cranial nerve functions were normal. Strength, sensory perception, and deep tendon reflexes of all extremities were normal. However, carotid bruits were audible bilaterally. Transthoracic echocardiography and Holter monitoring did not reveal any cardiac source of embolism.

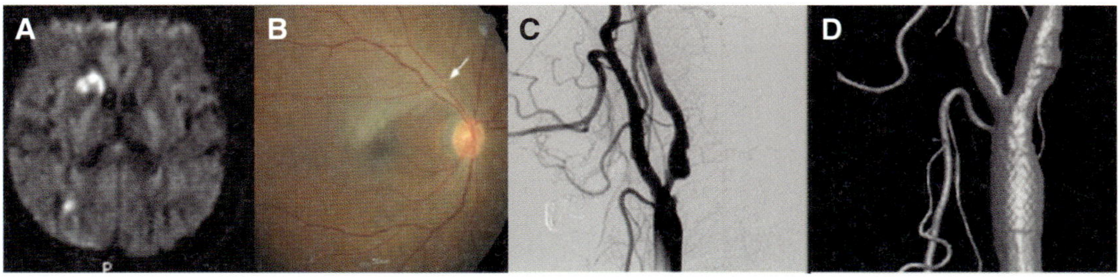

Brain MR-DWI (A) showed acute infarctions in the right caudate and parieto-occipital white matter. Funduscopic examination (B) revealed a "Hollenhorst plaque" at a retinal artery bifurcation, occluding the superior branch of the right retinal artery and causing ischemia of the superior half of the retina (arrow). Conventional angiography (C, D) showed bilateral proximal ICA stenoses (left: 50%, right: 80%). Although he had bilateral carotid stenosis, the right side was the only symptomatic side. Carotid stenting was performed in the right side successfully (D). However, immediately after the procedure, he presented confused state and drowsiness. DWI after the stenting showed multifocal acute ischemia in the right anterior circulation territory. Nevertheless, he was improved totally and discharged without further complication.

Carotid disease is the most frequent source for the retinal embolic arterial disease. Retinal emboli are most frequently located at arteriole bifurcation (B, arrow). They appear glistening and whitish. Recent guidelines suggest a significant benefit of endarterectomy for patients with a symptomatic stenosis > 50%. Nowadays, the result of endovascular approach and stenting is comparable to the result of endarterectomy.

• Case 144

A 68-year-old man presented with vertigo, which had developed 2 days earlier. The attacks of vertigo were transient lasting for 30 minutes, thus preventing him from walking. It recurred whenever he tried to walk. 2 years before the admission, he had experienced a sudden dysarthria to be diagnosed as a left basal ganglia infarction, and had taken aspirn thereafter. He had a history of hypertension. Examination revealed no gross abnormality in his cranial nerve functions, no nystagmus, no opthalmoplegia, and no paralysis of tongue protrusion. Strength and sensory perception of all limbs were normal. Hyperreflexia and Babinski sign were absent. Right-sided ataxia and right veering tendency were observed. Carotid bruit was inaudible. Transthoracic echocardiography showed no significant abnormality.

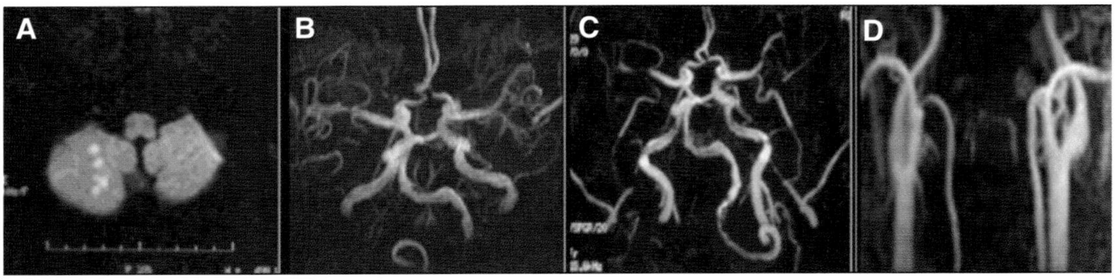

Brain MR-DWI (A) showed multiple acute infarctions in the right cerebellum. Brain MRA (B-D) showed no flow of right distal VA and tortous enlarged left VA. Combined antiplatelet agents were used for secondary prevention. He continued to improve and could walk without vertigo when he was discharged.

The stroke mechanism was in situ thrombosis of the right VA. Intracranial artery dolichoectasia may be asymptomatic, or may have clinical manifestations with acute onset (stroke or subarachnoid hemorrhage) or with chronic progressive presentation (cranial nerve palsy, compression of the midbrain, or obstructive hydrocephalus). Atherosclerosis is often present in the dolichoectatic arteries.[34] In this case, the atherosclerotic lesion of both VAs had progressed compared with the previous MRI.

• Case 145

A 66-year-old man visited our hospital presenting with dysarthria, dysphagia and left veering tendency. 1 day ago, after dinner he experienced sudden dizziness, left veering tendency, dysarthria, and dysphagia. These symptoms slowly progressed. There were no sensory symptoms. He had a previous stroke history 20 years ago presenting with a left-sided weakness and dysarthria. He had a hypertension and family history of stroke, but he did not have diabetes mellitus, hyperlipidemia and heart disease. He was a current 40-pack-year smoker. In neurologic examination, he showed normal mental status, but in cranial nerve examination, left facial palsy, dysarthria and dysphagia were observed. Motor power was MRC grade IV+ in his left side. Deep tendon reflex was increased and Babinski sign was positive on the left. In cerebellar function test, he revealed dysmetria in the left side and left veering tendency. ECG and Holter monitoring showed no remarkable findings except LVH.

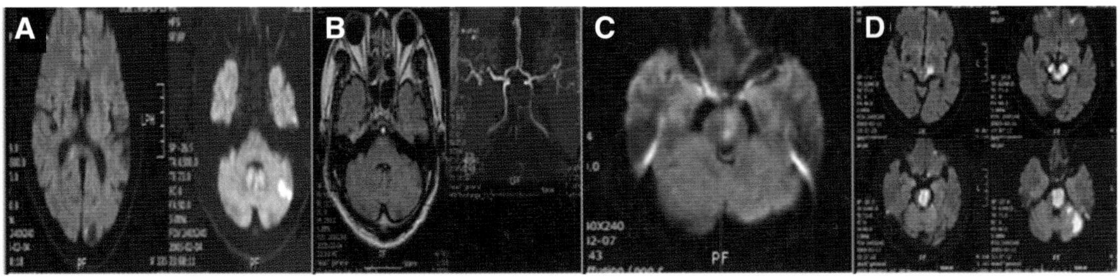

Brain MR-DWI (A) showed acute infarctions in the left cerebellum, left occipital lobe, right splenium and right parietal lobe. In the FLAIR and brain MRA (B), poor visualization of vertebrobasilar system and severe stenosis of the left distal ICA were observed. There was also an aneurysmal dilatation of BA secondary to thrombosis. We treated him with aspirin and clopidogrel. At the third day, a right-sided weakness developed and the medication was changed into heparin. At the seventh day, DWI showed multiple infarctions in pons, both midbrain and left thalamus (C, D). Consciousness level was decreased to semicomatose state and corneal reflex was absent in left side.

The stroke mechanisms of this patient were an artery to artery embolism from left VA and BA, and in situ thrombosis in the BA. Basilar artery thrombosis is a life threatening disease and can cause locked-in state or death. Acute infarctions within 6 hours are treatable with intraarterial thrombolysis. Evolving stroke with BA thrombosis should be treated aggressively. The anticoagulation should be considered and invasive procedure with thrombus aspiration and stent insertion is another option in grave situation.

• Case 146

A 63-year-old man with diabetes mellitus was hospitalized because of recurrent dizziness and transient diplopia, which was developed especially while he was pulling his cart. Neurological examination was normal except that his pulses of the left upper extremity were weak. Systolic BP measured on the left arm was lower by 30mmHg than that on the right arm. Transthoracic echocardiography and Holter monitoring did not reveal any cardiac source of embolism.

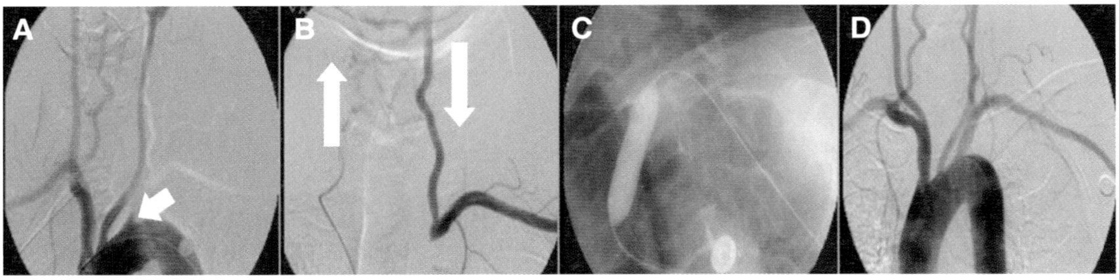

Conventional angiography (A, B) showed a severe stenosis of the left subclavian artery and vertebrobasilar steal phenomenon (arrows). A complete reversal of vertebral flow was provocated by quick deflation of BP cuff on the left arm (provocation test). The results of transcranial Doppler were normal, but provocation test with TCD showed the complete reversal of vertebral flow. Percutaneous transluminal angioplasty and stenting was done for the subclavian stenosis (C, D). After then, the reversal of vertebral blood flow was not demonstrated on the TCD. The dizziness or diplopia has not recurred any more.

Subclavian steal syndrome refers to a clinically significant vertebrobasilar insufficiency resulting from a reversal of blood flow through the VA due to occlusion or stenosis of the proximal subclavian artery. Percutaneous intravascular intervention can be a good therapeutic method for subclavian steal syndrome.

• Case 147

A 59-year-old, right-handed man presented with a sudden onset of left-sided weakness, which had been developed 2 days prior to visit. When he visited our hospital, the weakness was much improved. He had diabetes mellitus, hypercholesterolemia and hypertension with regular medication. He was alert and neglect was absent. His speech was slightly dysarthric. There was no objective abnormality in the motor and sensory examination. Transthoracic echocardiography and Holter monitoring did not reveal any cardiac source of embolism. HbA1c was 8.3%. Total cholesterolemia was 288mg/dL.

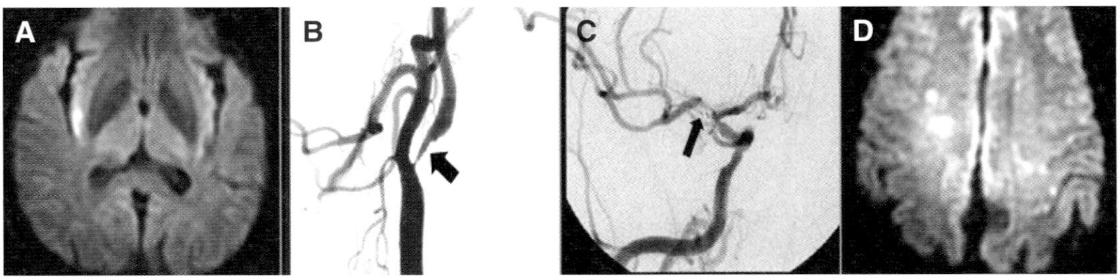

Brain MR-DWI (A) showed an acute infarction in the right insular cortex. Conventional angiography (B, C) showed severe stenoses in the left proximal ICA and right proximal M1 (arrows). He was treated with dual antiplatelet agents, statin and insulin. About 3 weeks after admission, angioplasty and stent insertion for the left proximal ICA stenosis were performed under a protective device. During post-stent angioplasty, systolic BP fell down to about 60mmHg for a few minutes and right-sided weakness and aphasia were detected. Pharmacological elevation of BP was done shortly after that. Follow-up DWI after stenting in the left proximal ICA showed acute infarctions in both hemispheres (D).

Lesion in the right insular cortex was thought to result from an artery to artery embolism from the proximal ICA or MCA. However, the mechanism of stroke in the bilateral borderzone after angioplasty was low-flow because there was an episode of hypotension and lesions involve borderzones of both hemispheres. Careful intervention should be performed for patients with proximal ICA disease combined with tandem or contra-lateral lesions.

• Case 148

A 48-year-old right-handed man presented with a left-sided weakness, which had been developed 4 days before admission. Dysarthria and left side hypesthesia was associated. 2 days after admission in the local hospital, he showed irritable behavior and the left-sided weakness was aggravated. He was transferred to our hospital. 20 years before, he had been diagnosed as hypertension, but he did not take any medication. His mental status was alert. Cranial nerve examination showed left visual field defect, and left central-type facial palsy. Motor power was MRC grade I in the upper extremity and III in the lower extremity. Sensory system revealed left hypesthesia. Echocardiography revealed no abnormality except concentric LVH.

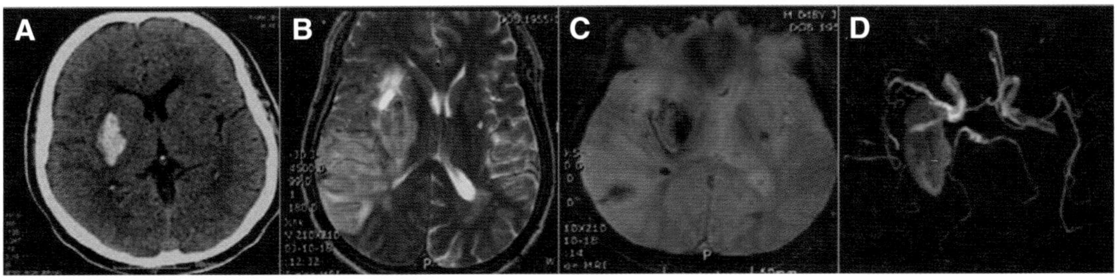

Initial brain CT (A) showed an acute hemorrhage in the right basal ganglia. Follow-up brain MRI (B, C) showed a hemorrhagic infarction in the right MCA. Brain MRA (D) showed no significant stenoocclusive lesions. Antiplatelet agent was not given. His clinical state was stationary. After acute management and rehabilitation, he was discharged.

Initially, he showed a right basal ganglia hemorrhage. 2 days after, a new right MCA territorial hemorrhagic infarction occurred. MR angiography showed a vascular displacement without stenoocclusive lesion due to hemorrhage. Initial stroke may be due to hypertensive hemorrhage because of chronic hypertension and microangiopathy. Second event may be due to a cardioembolism with no documented source. Therapeutic approach such as BP control should be carefully done in this situation.

• Case 149

A 74-year-old man presented with a sudden left-sided weakness, which had been developed 2 hours before admission. Medical history included hypertension with regular treatment. He was a current smoker of 50 packyears. He was slightly drowsy, but showed anosognosia and neglect to the left side. Cranial nerve examination showed right gaze preponderance and left homonymous hemianopsia. Left central-type facial palsy, hypesthesia and dysarthria were evident. The motor power of the left side was MRC grade I. The sensory examination revealed left side hypesthesia. The toe sign of the left side was extensor. The carotid and ophthalmic bruits were inaudible. Transthoracic echocardiography and Holter monitoring did not reveal any cardiac source of embolism.

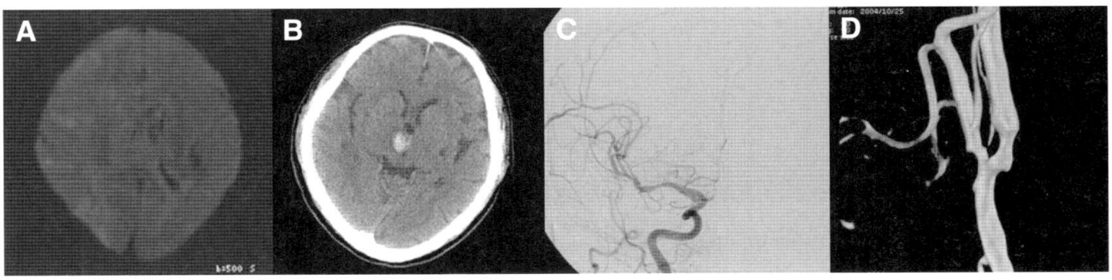

He visited our hospital 2 hours after the symptom onset. Initial brain CT revealed no abnormal findings. So thrombolysis with intravenous rt-PA was done. After thrombolysis, his mental status became alert, but other neurologic deficits were stationary. Brain MR-DWI (A) showed acute infarctions in the right MCA territory. Follow-up brain CT after intravenous thrombolysis (B), an intraventricular hemorrhage was developed in the third ventricle. TFCA (C, D) showed intact intracranial arteries but a moderate stenosis in the right proximal ICA. 1 day after, he was treated with antiplatelet agent. His symptoms slowly improved.

The MCA infarction in this patient was due to an artery to artery embolism from the right proximal ICA. Because the degree of ICA stenosis was not so severe but symptomatic, TFCA and angioplasty should be planned in this patient. CT scan after thrombolysis showed a 3rd ventricular hemorrhage without further neurologic deterioration.

• Case 150

A 54-year-old woman developed a sudden left-sided weakness and felt drowsy mentality 2 hours before visiting emergency department. She had a history of atrial fibrillation and hypertension and had been treated with aspirin. Examination showed drowsy mentality and hemineglect on the left side. She also showed left central facial palsy, left facial hypethesia, and dysarthria. Strength in her left side was MRC grade II. All sensory modalities were diminished in her left side. Hyperreflexia and bilateral Babinski signs were present. NIHSS at admission was 15.

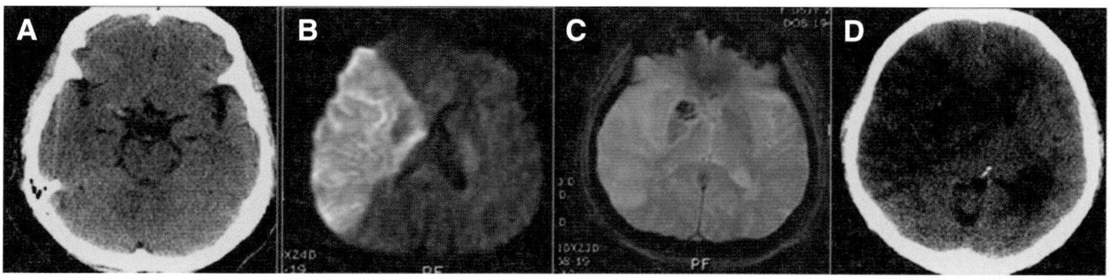

Initial Brain CT (A) showed so-called, dense MCA sign in the proximal MCA. The rt-PA was administered at 2.5 hours after symptom onset, but neurologic deficit was not improved. Brain MR-DWI (B) showed an acute infarction involving the entire right MCA territory. This patient developed a whole territorial infarction of the right MCA and a hemorrhagic transformation in the basal ganglia without improvement despite the intraarterial thrombolysis (C, D). Although she had atrial fibrillation, large size infarction and hemorrhagic transformation limited anticoagulation therapy. NIHSS at discharge was 12.

This patient developed a whole territorial infarction of the right MCA. This patient had a high risk factor for cardioembolic stroke. The emboli manifesting as a dense MCA sign often locate from the distal ICA (T-portion), and as in this case, large emboli are often resistant to intravenous thrombolysis therapy. As in this patient, the large territorial infarction gives us the rationale to perform craniectomy when there is continuing deterioration.

• Case 151

A 68-year-old man was admitted for angiographic evaluation. He had a medical history of diabetes mellitus for 20 years which was well-controlled. 18 months before, cerebral angioplasty and stent insertion had been done because of severe stenosis in the cavernous portion of the left ICA and symptomatic lesion in the corresponding area. In the follow-up brain MRA, we detected an increased flow defect in the area of stent insertion. However, patent flow in the cavernous ICA was confirmed on the subsequent CT angiography.

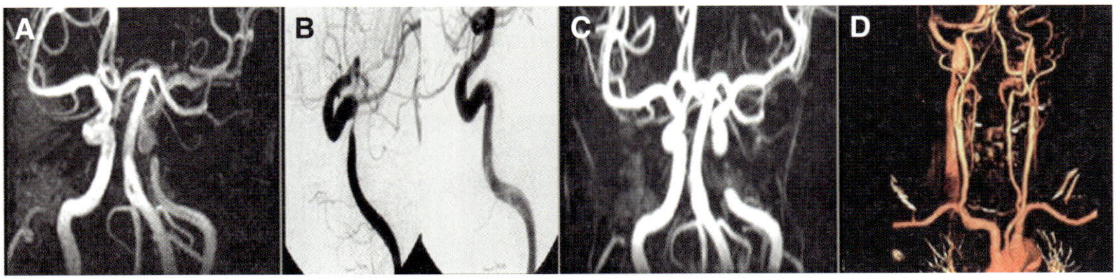

Brain MRA (A) revealed a significant stenosis of the proximal cavernous portion of the ICA. Cerebral angioplasty and stent insertion (B) for this lesion were done because of a symptomatic severe stenosis. Follow-up brain MRA (C) showed no flow in the proximal cavernous segment of left ICA possibly due to stent artifact. However, CT angiography (D) could identify a patent flow in the cavernous ICA. We maintained his medication of aspirin and clopidogrel.

Metallic stents cause susceptibility and radiofrequency artifacts on MR images, which have not allowed for a complete visualization of the stent lumen by MRA. CT angiography would be more helpful to evaluate the stent patency.

• Case 152

A 42-year-old man with headache visited emergency room. He had complained of insidious headache and dizziness for a few days, and had visited a local hospital. Hypoxemia and irregular respiratory pattern were detected. He was transferred to our hospital after ICU care for 2 days. 13 years before admission, he had undertaken a surgical clipping for Acom and MCA aneurysm. After this operation, right MCA infarct had been developed. Also he had diabetes mellitus, hypertension and smoking history of 60 packyears. He was drowsy and irritable but orientation was intact. All of the brainstem reflexes were normal. There was no asymmetry of facial expression or limb movement. TFCA was done, but no evidence of SAH was found. Echocardiogram was not done.

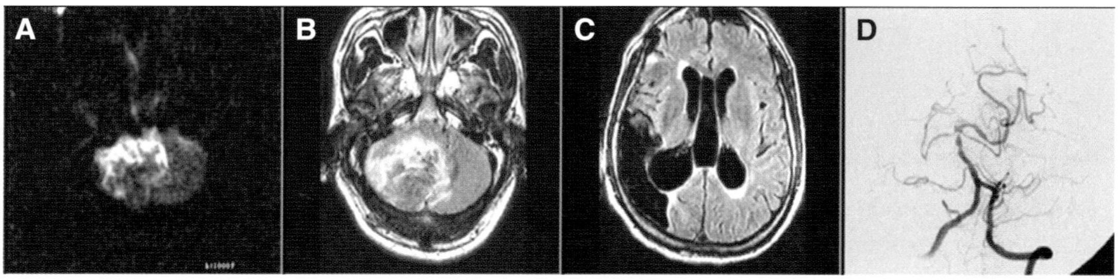

MRI (A, B) showed an acute infarct with hemorrhagic conversion in the right PICA territory with brainstem compression. He was taken care of in ICU due to brainstem compression and treated with mannitol and an antiplatelet agent under a mechanical ventilator. Some degree of hydrocephalus was accompanied (C) but his mentality and respiration improved slowly. Conventional angiography (D) showed an occlusion of the right PICA and focal stenoses of BA and both proximal PCAs. Only mild dizziness was left when he was discharged.

There was an infarction with hemorrhagic conversion in the whole PICA territory. There were multiple stenoses in the vertebrobasilar artery. Although the evaluation for embolism was incomplete, the probable mechanism of stroke was in situ thrombosis, but an artery to artery embolism of the right VA could not be excluded. Subsequent edema formation from the initial infarct becomes space occupying within the posterior fossa, leading to brainstem compression, hydrocephalus, cardiorespiratory complications, coma, and death. This complication occurs in 10-25% of patients, peaking on the third day after the infarction, although it can occur any time within the first week.[35]

• Case 153

3 days before admission, 60-year-old man had developed a right-sided weakness and global aphasia. At that time he had visited a local hospital. His symptoms were more aggravated and he was transferred to our hospital. His mental state was slightly drowsy. He showed global aphasia, left gaze preponderance, and right homonymous hemianopsia. And he showed right central-type facial palsy, right hemiplegia, and hypesthesia. Deep tendon reflex showed hyperreflexia in the right side. His past medical history showed old myocardial infarction. Transthoracic echocardiography revealed 35-40% of ejection fraction and anteroseptal and apical akinesia.

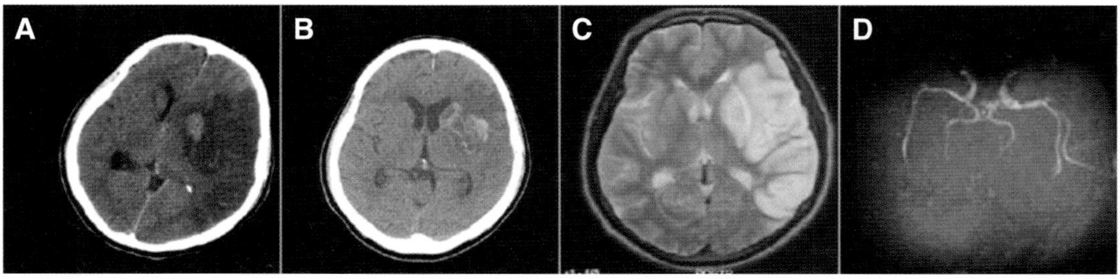

Brain CT (A) revealed a left MCA infarction with hemorrhagic conversion and mass effect. Mannitol and aspirin was started. 2 weeks later, we added low-dose warfarin on aspirin after follow-up CT (B) and MRI (C). Brain MRA (D) showed an incomplete filling of the left MCA.

The stroke mechanism was a cardioembolism, and anticoagulants could be administered after evaluation of the size of infarction and degree of hemorrhagic transformation at follow-up MRI or CT.

• Case 154

A 68-year-old woman was admitted because of a sudden left-sided weakness. 10 years before admission, he had suffered from hypertension and diabetes mellitus, and taken regular medicine. He had no history of heart disease or previous stroke. She was alert and oriented with intact cognitive function. There was no motor or visual neglect on the left side. Cranial nerve examinations were normal except for mild dysarthria. His left upper extremity was weak (MRC grade IV-). Sensory examination showed no abnormal findings. Ataxia, tremor and gait abnormality were not noted. Transthoracic echocardiography and Holter monitoring did not reveal any cardiac source of embolism.

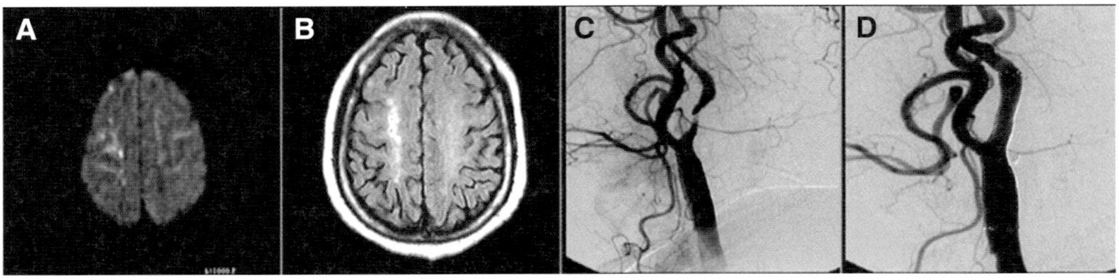

MRI (A, B) showed multiple punctate lesions in the right centrum semiovale. Conventional angiography (C) showed a severe stenosis in the right proximal ICA, but with relatively intact intracranial vessel. TCD could detect several spontaneous microembolic signals during the right MCA monitoring. He was treated with dual antiplatelet agents. His neurological symptoms improved fully. With an interval of 1 month after the symptom onset, stent insertion was performed in the right proximal ICA without complication (D). On the follow-up TCD, there were no further microembolic signals.

The lesions were located mainly in the internal borderzone. The putative stroke mechanism was an artery to artery embolism from the proximal ICA. TCD could detect microembolic signals, suggestive of vulnerable plaque on the proximal vessels. Carotid stenting could stabilize unstable plaque as well as improve hemodynamic status.

• Case 155

A 62-year-old man visited emergency department with a right hand weakness and numbness. 2 hours before the admission, he had experienced a transient right hand weakness and numbness. The symptoms were totally disappeared when he visit the hospital. He had a history of hypercholesterolemia without hypertension and diabetes mellitus. Neurologic examination showed no abnormality at the admission. No bruit was audible on his neck. Transthoracic echocardiography and Holter monitoring did not reveal any cardiac source of embolism.

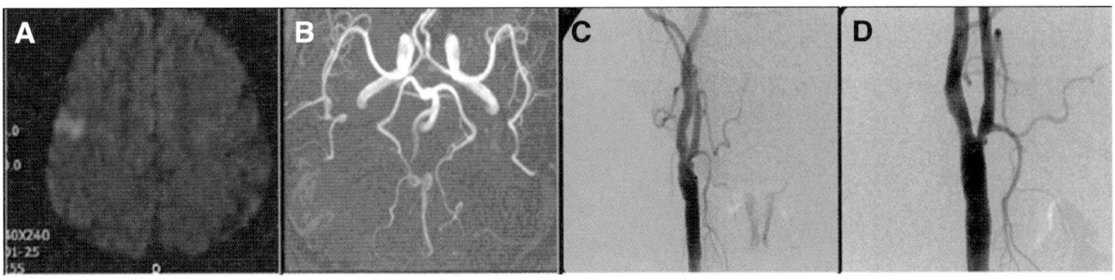

Brain MR-DWI (A, B) showed a focal acute infarction in the right frontal cortical area. Brain MRA (B) showed no significant abnormality. Conventional angiography (C) identified an atheromatous plaque with ulceration at the right distal CCA and proximal ICA with mild stenosis. The degree of stenosis was about 40%. He received stent placement in the right proximal ICA and distal CCA, without any neurologic complication (D). He was discharged with antiplatelet agent and statin.

Atherosclerotic plaque in the right CCA bifurcation fired emboli to the right frontal cortical area. Although the degree of stenosis was low, angioplasty was tried because the stenosis was obviously symptomatic one.

• Case 156

A 55-year-old man was admitted because of dyspnea on exertion, and given pacemaker at cardiology. 10 days after admission, he presented with dizziness and altered mentality. He had atrial fibrillation and was a 40-pack-year ex-smoker, but did not have hypertension and diabetes mellitus. He also had a previous stroke history of left hemiparesis and dysarthria 5 months ago. On neurologic examination, his mental status was drowsy and verbal response was decreased. Vestibuloocular reflex and corneal reflex were intact. Motor power was MRC grade III in four extremities. Deep tendon reflex was preserved. ECG showed atrial fibrillation. Echocardiogram showed dilated LV cavity size and severely depressed systolic function with estimated ejection fraction 20-25%.

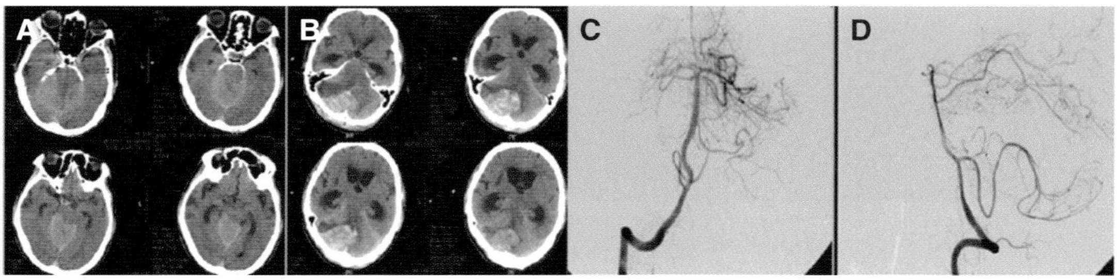

Brain MRI couldn't be performed due to pacemaker. We checked brain CT and TFCA. Brain CT (A) revealed a massive infarction in posterior fossa, cerebellum and brainstem with upward transtentorial herniation. After 3 days, follow-up brain CT (B) was checked and there was a hemorrhagic transformation in the right cerebellum, and obstructive hydrocephalus. Conventional angiography (C, D) demonstrated an absent opacification of the right PICA and a delayed contrast circulation in the left PICA. Bilateral cerebellar infarctions were thought to be lesions lasing over 24 hours. We planned decompression surgery due to brainstem compression and obstructive hydrocephalus but the procedure could not be done by the family members' objection. The patient fell to brain death and died of cardiac arrest.

The stroke mechanism of this patient was a cardioembolism. Large cerebellar infarction can cause brainstem compression and hydrocephalus.[35] Selective surgery with IICP control can rescue the patient. TFCA revealed delayed or blocked circulation of both PICAs about 1 or 2 days after ischemic stroke.

• Case 157

A 73-year-old man presented with a transient left-sided weakness. He had a history of diabetes mellitus and hypercholesterolemia, which were well-controlled, and angina pectoris 3 years ago. He was a 70-pack-year current smoker. 1 day before admission, he had felt a sudden left limb weakness and dysarthria in the middle of lunch, but the symptoms disappeared in 30 minutes. Neurologic examination was entirely normal. Transthoracic echocardiography and Holter monitoring did not reveal any cardiac source of embolism.

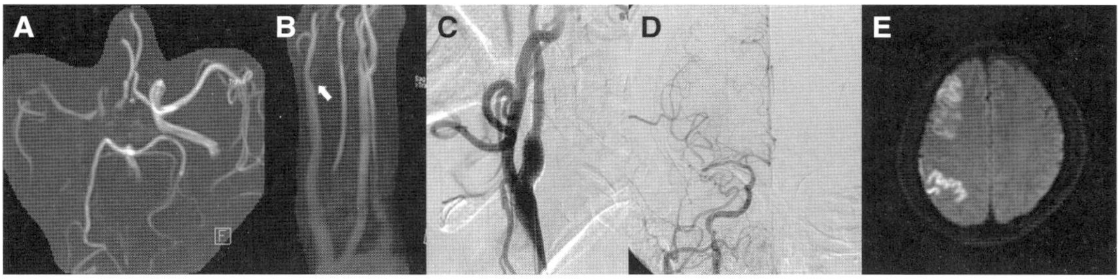

Brain MR-DWI revealed an acute infarct in the right MCA, superior division territory. MRA (A, B) showed a complete occlusion of the right ICA at the proximal portion (arrow). We penetrated ICA thrombus with microcatheter, made ballooning within the thrombus with distal protective device, and deployed stent in the proximal ICA (C). The ICA was recanalyzed and the MCA flow was increased after stent insertion. No thrombotic material was detected in the protective device. However, severe stenosis in right superior division was also identified (D). After stenting, he showed asomatognosia in the right limb and gaze preponderance to the left side. Subsequent DWI revealed new acute infarctions in the right frontal lobe and parietal lobe (E). We managed him with aspirin, clopidogrel, and atorvastatin. The gaze preponderance and neglect improved at discharge, but mild frontal lobe dysfunction (perseveration) was left.

Balloon angioplasty and stenting may be feasible and effective in an acute occlusion of the proximal ICA. However, thromboembolic events can frequently occur during procedures. The embolic protection device is likely to be helpful. His recurrent TIA and post-stenting infarction are thought to be due to thromboembolism from the proximal ICA to MCA division.

• Case 158

A 38-year-old man was admitted presenting with aphasia. 1 day before admission during conversation, a global aphasia had developed suddenly. He had difficulty in comprehension and expression. Mild dysarthria was associated. There was no headache, nausea or vomiting. Stroke risk factors such as diabetes mellitus, hypertension, smoking and cardiac disease were absent. On neurological examination, he showed a mild sensory-motor aphasia and other neurologic exams were normal. In laboratory tests, abnormal findings were not observed. ECG and echocardiography were normal.

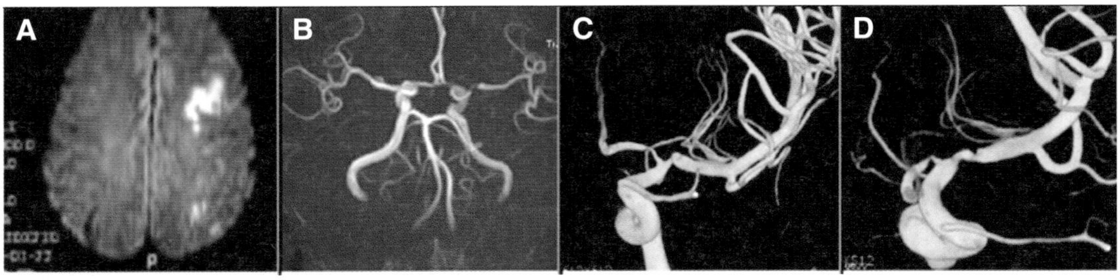

Brain MR-DWI (A) showed multifocal small acute infarctions in the left posterior border zone and the left frontal lobe. Brain MRA (B) showed severe stenoses in the left proximal A1 and M1. Brain SPECT showed a decreased vascular reserve in the left MCA territory. Primary angioplasty was done for this lesion (C, D). Aphasia improved slowly and he was discharged with reservation of follow-up conventional cerebral angiography.

The stroke mechanism of this patient was an artery to artery embolism from stenotic portion of left M1. Thus, a medical therapy targeting for unstable atherosclerosis and endothelial dysfunction was the best option. We should cautiously consider angioplasty/stenting in the low flow condition associated with the intracranial artery stenosis. TCD and CTA follow-up are needed with a careful observation of clinical course.

• Case 159

A 69-year-old man was admitted because of a gangrenous change of right great toe. He had a history of diabetes mellitus and hypertension without medications. During workup for newly detected atherosclerosis obliterans, on carotid Doppler, abnormal findings were incidentally detected. He was transferred to department of neurology. On neurologic examination, there were no remarkable findings. Transthoracic echocardiography and Holter monitoring did not reveal any cardiac source of embolism.

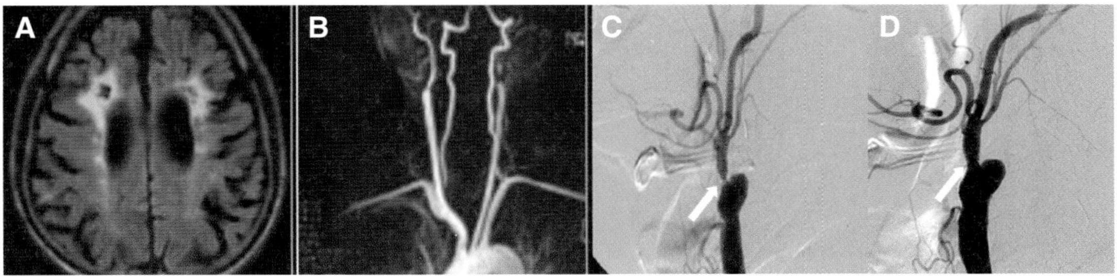

MRI (A) showed no evidence of acute infarct except chronic periventricular white matter changes with small infarcts. Brain MRA (B) and conventional angiography (C) revealed occlusion of both proximal ICA and severe stenosis of both ECA. We performed both ECA stent (D) and treated him with aspirin and clopidogrel.

As we supposed that a partial recovery of the blood flow through both ECAs can improve his hemodynamic status, we performed stent insertion in both ECAs. In ASO patients, stenosis or occlusion of ICA or ECA are common, so carotid Doppler or brain MRA is needed if possible. However, the efficacy and long-term patency of ECA stent remain to be followed in this case.

• Case 160

A 67-year-old man was admitted because of both ICA stenoses. 5 months before admission, incidental stenosis of both proximal ICA was detected on carotid Doppler. He had a history of hypertension and diabetes mellitus. There were no previous stroke history and hyperlipidemia. Neurologic examination was normal except both carotid bruits. HbA1c was 10.1%. ECG and echocardiography were normal. Carotid Doppler showed stenoses of bilateral proximal ICA (right < 35%, Left < 55%).

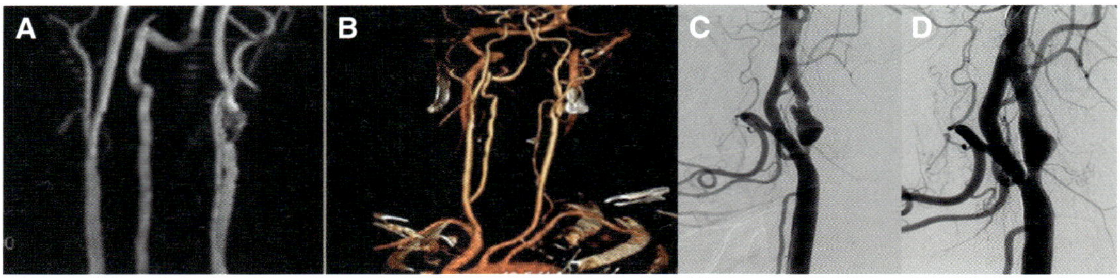

Brain MRI showed small silent ischemic lesions in the left PVWM. Brain MRA (A) and CT angiography (B) showed severe stenoses with ulceration in the proximal portion of both ICAs. Angioplasty with stent insertion was done in the left proximal ICA (C, D). After angioplasty, systolic BP was dropped from 130 to 80mmHg. We treated him with intravenous dopamine. He also showed orthostatic hypotension. 1 day after angioplasty, heart rate was decreased to a 48/min. BP and heart rate recovered over a few days.

Hypotension and bradycardia after carotid artery stenting is relatively common, especially in case that carotid lesion involves a carotid bulb. There was a report that hypotension resolve within 2 days.[36] Inotropic agents can be used during the hypotensive period.

• Case 161

A 69-year-old right-handed man was referred for the right-sided weakness. He had a medical history of hypertension, which was poorly controlled, but did not have any other stroke risk factors. 3 days prior to the admission, he had suffered a sudden right-sided weakness (MRC grade II), and could not understand the conversation. He was given a treatment of intra-arterial thrombolysis on the left proximal ICA and anticoagulant at a local hospital. He had severe steno-occlusive lesions in bilateral proximal ICA, and was transferred to our hospital for further management. The heart beat was regular, but a high pitch bruit was heard in the right carotid artery. He could obey to two step commands, and had a weakness (MRC grade IV) in the right side. Transthoracic echocardiography and Holter monitoring did not reveal any cardiac source of embolism.

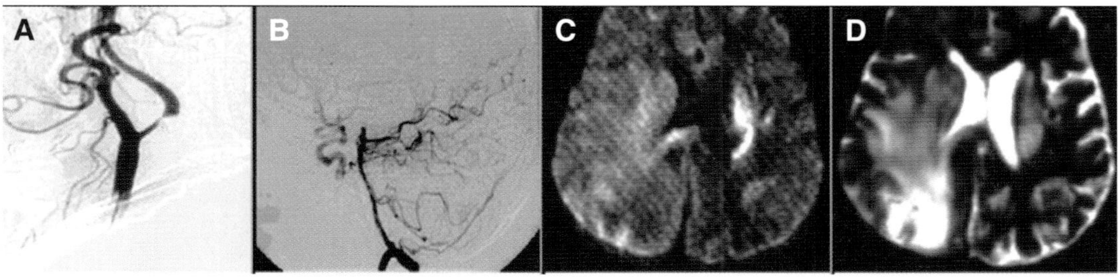

Conventional angiography showed a severe stenosis in the right proximal ICA (A) and a complete occlusion of the left proximal ICA while left MCA and distal ICA was supplied through trigeminal artery. CEA was successfully done in the right side after 4 weeks of the stroke onset. He did not complain any symptoms after endarterectomy for a few days. On the postop 2 days, however, he became drowsy and disoriented showing right gaze preponderance and left limb weakness as well as several generalized tonic clonic seizure attacks with left versive movement. Brain MR-DWI (C, D) showed diffuse high signal intensity in the right MCA territory without ADC decrease. EEG showed PLEDs in the right hemisphere. We also could see an increased flow velocity in the right ICA, MCA, and ACA on TCD while the BP was well-controlled.

The hyperperfusion syndrome is characterized by headache, seizure, and focal neurologic deficit several days after CEA or angioplasty, and often predisposed by preoperative loss of cerebral autoregulation before the correction of high grade carotid stenosis. The immediate MRI image indicated high signal intensity in the right MCA territory, but the ADC was not decreased in the same territory representing vasogenic edema.

• Case 162

A 76-year-old man presented with agitation. 5 years prior to visit, he had been diagnosed with right PCA infarction due to a sudden onset of visual field defect. 6 months before, stenoses of both proximal ICA were detected on the follow-up brain MRA. He underwent angioplasty and stent insertion on the left side and received same procedure on the other side 1 month later. The last procedure was complicated with multiple right MCA infarctions which resulted in mild left-sided weakness. After discharge, he became restless and sleepless of which onset was uncertain. He also had a coronary artery disease and his medication included clopidogrel. He was alert and orientation was intact. No behavioral abnormality was found during the examination. Dressing apraxia and left visual field defect which had resulted from the previous stroke was found. Left motor power was weak but not worse than before. Transthoracic echocardiography did not reveal any source of embolism.

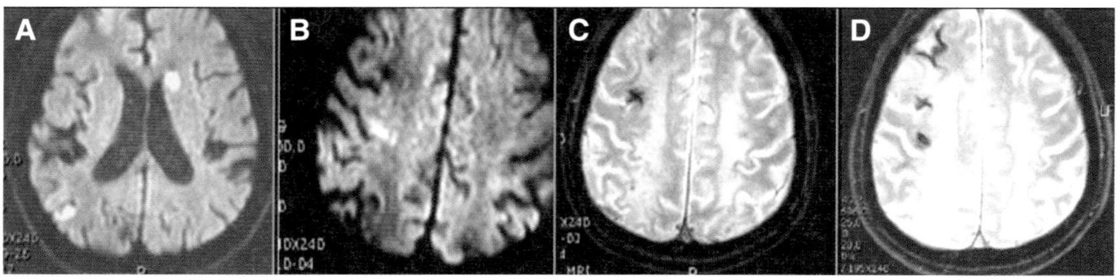

Brain MR-DWI (A, B) showed acute infarctions in the left caudate, right frontal and parieto-occipital lobe. GRE images (C, D) indicated the increased extent of microhemorrhage. He was treated with clopidogrel with aspirin. His symptom was slightly improved.

There were multiple embolic events after stenting. There was no in-stent thrombosis in both proximal ICAs. Multiple microbleeds were also demonstrated in some areas suggesting embolizations. Since there were no cardioembolic sources, we gave him dual antiplatelet agents instead of anticoagulant.

• Case 163

A 69-year-old man presented with a left-sided weakness and numbness. The symptoms were suddenly developed 2 hours prior to visit. He had hypertension and ischemic heart disease with CABG at the age of 45 years and percutaneous intervention at the age of 67 years. He had taken dual antiplatelet agents since that time.

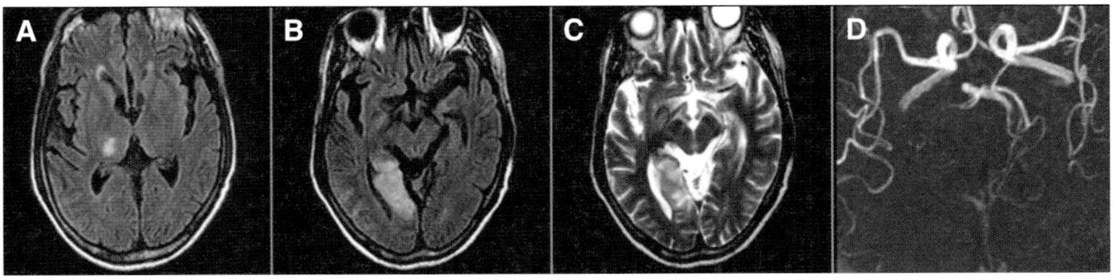

MRI (A-C) showed acute ischemic infarctions in the right posterior medial temporooccipital lobe and right thalamus corresponding to right PCA territory. Brain MRA (D) showed an occlusion of the right PCA. He was treated with an anticoagulant. On the ninth day after onset, synkinesia was detected. When he voluntarily moved the big toe on the paretic side, the 2nd finger also moved simultaneously tuned to flexion and extension on the same side.

The mechanism of stroke on the unilateral PCA territory is mostly an embolism as this patient. Imitative ipsilateral limb movements (i.e., arm levitation when attempting to lift the leg) have rarely been mentioned in the literature, and the anatomic correlate of such unusual movements is unknown.[37] Disruption of corticothalamic motor inhibitory pathways may be the mechanism. Hypometabolism of this inhibitory motor pathway has already been implicated in spontaneous arm levitation of patients with corticobasal ganglionic degeneration.[38]

• Case 164

A 51-year-old right-handed woman presented with dysarthria and left leg weakness, which was developed 4 days ago. She had suffered a right MCA infarction 9 years before, and taken aspirin since that time. Recent left motor power had been measured as MRC grade III in arm and grade IV+ in leg. She had congestive heart failure and end stage renal disease with regular hemodialysis. She was alert and oriented, but showed a spastic-type dysarthria and an aggravated left lower extremity weakness (MRC grade III). However, she had no deteriorating body sense in the left limb. There was no motor weakness in the right side, either. Electrocardiography showed left ventricular hypertrophy with arrhythmia.

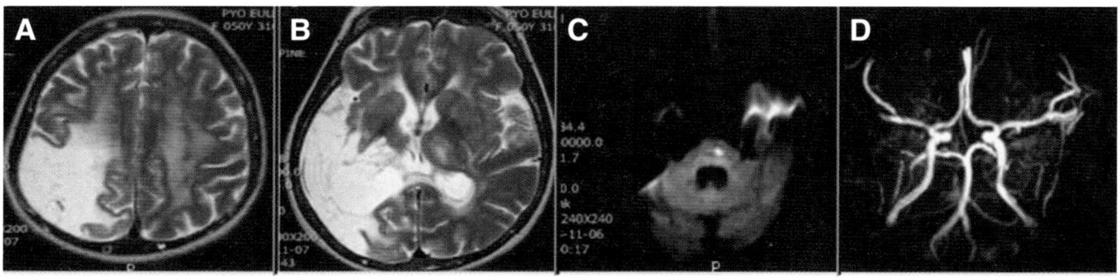

Brain MRI (A, B) showed a massive cerebromalacia in the right temporo-occipital lobe associated with wallerian degeneration of the right cerebral peduncle. There was also severe small vessel disease and multiple microbleeds. MR-DWI (C) showed an acute infarction in the left pons. Brain MRA (D) identified an occlusion of the inferior division of right MCA. She was treated with antiplatelet combination of aspirin and clopidogrel, and had better motor function in the right leg to be able to walk with a cane.

There was an old large infarction with massive cerebromalacia in the right MCA territory involving motor cortex and corona radiata. MR-DWI revealed a small high signal intensity lesion in the left pons, which was proved to be an acute infarction in ADC map. This patient did not complain of any right motor dysfunction. Although by chance the lesion was too small to produce damage to the crossed corticospinal tract, it is more likely that the infarction induces direct damage to the uncrossed corticospinal tract itself, in a functionally reorganized motor tract from the previous stroke.

• Case 165

A 65-year-old, right-handed man presented with a sudden onset of language disturbance. 15 years prior to visit, he had been diagnosed with left MCA infarction due to sensory aphasia. His language function had been improved much so that he could have a simple conversation with his family. 2 days prior to admission, he could not understand words at all but he could speak with fluency. He had diabetes mellitus, hypertension and hyperlipidemia. He had undergone off-pump CABG due to angina 2 years before. His medication included clopidogrel. He was alert, but typical sensory aphasia was detected. Right homonymous hemianopsia was also detected, which had resulted from the previous stroke. Motor power and sensory were normal. Transthoracic echocardiography did not reveal any source of embolism.

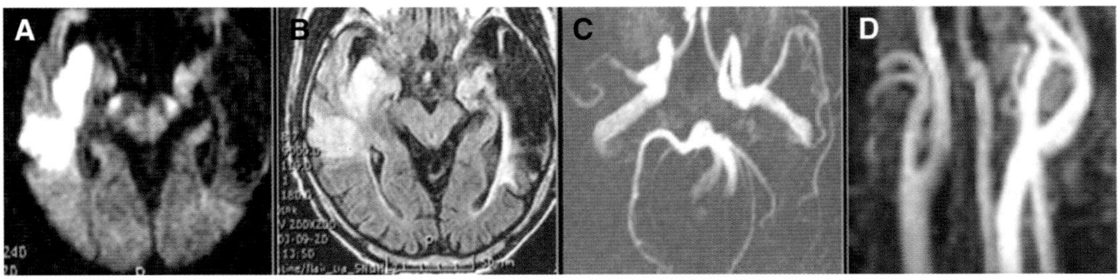

Brain MR-DWI (A) showed an acute infarction in the right MCA inferior division, and FLAIR image (B) showed a cerebromalacia in the left MCA inferior division. Brain MRA (C, D) showed a total occlusion of the right M1 and no significant stenosis in the neck vessels. Intermittently, he showed aggressive behaviors for several days. When discharged, aphasia was not improved and aggressive behavior disappeared.

This is a case of sensory aphasia aggravated by right temporal lobe lesion after previous left temporal lobe infarction. When a specific function is lost by a specific cerebral lesion, other intact cerebral brain area, which can be opposite side, takes over the lost function (functional reorganization) for recovery according to the functional takeover theory.[39]

• Case 166

A 64-year-old right-handed woman came to emergency room for a left-sided weakness. She had a history of hypertension, which was well-controlled. She had suffered a right corona radiata infarction 9 years before and right thalamic hemorrhage 3 months before, but walked by herself with a cane thereafter. 2 days prior to admission, she realized aggravated left limb weakness on awakening. She also felt mild dysarthria and facial weakness in the left side, which had not been noticed in previous stroke events. Neurologic examination revealed central-type facial palsy and limb weakness (MRC grade III) in the left side with more severe weakness in distal muscle. However, there was neither sensory change in both sides nor newly developed right weakness.

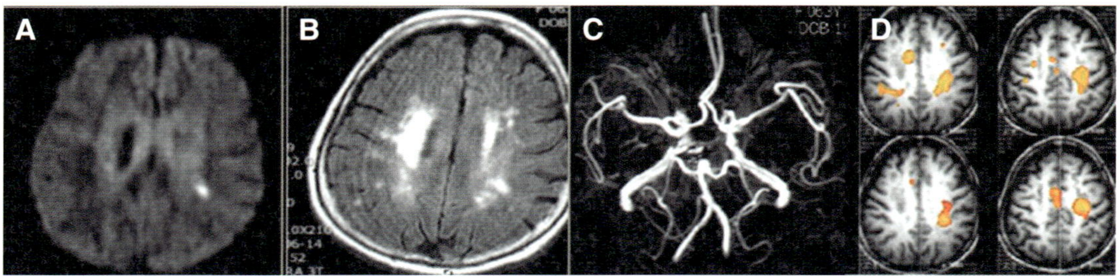

MRI (A, B) showed acute infarction in the left posterior periventricular corona radiata and old infarction in the right corona radiata. Brain MRA (C) showed no significant stenoocclusive lesions. The functional MRI 2 weeks later showed more activation of the left motor cortex than the right motor cortex by left hand grip (upper row of D), and activation of the left motor cortex only by a right hand grip (lower row of D). She could lift her arm and walk with a cane, but had difficult gripping the left hand 1 month later.

This rare case could provide obvious evidences about the important role of cortical reorganization within the motor areas of the unaffected hemisphere for stroke recovery. Generally, contralesional activation is considered to be useful in the acute/subacute stage, but its relative contribution would decline as recovery proceeds.[40] Nevertheless, we often see the contralateral hemisphere functions after the one-sided brain damage such as stroke.

• Case 167

A 43-year-old right-handed man presented with a sudden left limb weakness. 20 days prior to visit, he had felt a sudden left limb weakness with numbness, and heard to have a cerebral infarction from a doctor, but the symptoms had been improved to disappear until recently. On the day of admission, he experienced newly developed left limb weakness and visited emergency room. He had a medical history of hypertension with retinopathy and was an ex-smoker who had quitted 10 years before. Neurologic examination revealed mild left-sided weakness and hypesthesia involving face and limbs. The weakness was more severe in the leg (MRC grade IV-) than the arm (MRC grade IV+). Echocardiography and ECG did not show any abnormal finding.

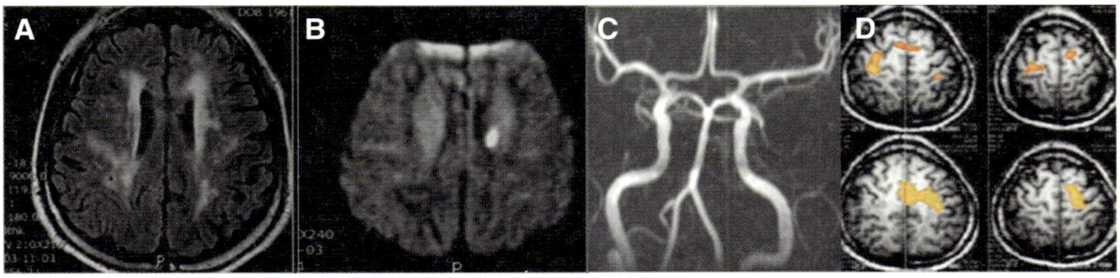

MRI (A, B) showed a severe small vessel disease in bilateral hemispheres and an acute infarction in the left corona radiata. Brain MRA (C) showed no significant stenoocclusive lesions. The functional MRI after 2 weeks indicated an activation of both motor cortices by left hand grip (upper row of D) and activation of left motor cortex by right hand grip (lower row of D). He was given aspirin medication, and discharged without neurologic deficit 2 weeks later.

Although correlations between recovery and the amount of activation have not been reported as yet, these would be simply explained by less severe lesion in the right corona radiata requiring less contralesional activation. And, the premotor area, which was more activated in this patient, was thought to be of some importance for the restoration of motor functions.

REFERENCES

1. Adams HP Jr, Bendixen BH, Kappelle LJ, Biller J, Love BB, Gordon DL, Marsh EE 3rd. Classification of Subtype of Acute Ischemic Stroke: Definitions for Use in a Multicenter Clinical Trial. TOAST. Trial of Org 10172 in Acute Stroke Treatment. Stroke, 1993: 24; 35-41.
2. Ferro JM. Cardioembolic Stroke: An Update. Lancet Neurol, 2003: 2; 177-188.
3. Kitchens GS. Thrombophilia and Thrombosis in Unusual Sities. In RW Colman, J Hirsh, VJ Marder, et al. (eds), Hemostasis and Thrombosis: Basic Principles and Clinical Practice (3rd ed). Philadelphia: Lippincott-Raven, 1994: 1255-1273.
4. Diagnosis and Management of Cerebral Vasculitis. In HP Adams Jr (ed), Handbook of Cerebrovascular Diseases. New York: Marcel Dekker, 1993: 549-567.
5. Leys D, Mounier-Vehier F, Lavenu I, Rondepierre P, Pruvo JP. Anterior Choroidal Artery Territory Infarcts. Study of Presumed Mechanisms. Stroke, 1994: 25; 837-842.
6. Roh JK, Kang DW, Lee SH, Yoon BW, Chang KH. Significance of Acute Multiple Brain Infarction on Diffusion-Weighted Imaging. Stroke, 2000: 31; 688-694.
7. Nicolai A, Lazzarino LG, Biasutti E. Large Striatocapsular Infarcts: Clinical Features and Risk Factors. J Neurol, 1996: 243; 44-50.
8. Ye BS, Kim YD, Nam HS, Lee HS, Nam CM, Heo JH. Clinical Manifestations of Cerebellar Infarction According to Specific Lobular Involvement. Cerebellum, 2010: 9; 571-579.
9. Kameda W, Kawanami T, Kurita K, Daimon M, Kayama T, Hosoya T, Kato T; Study Group of the Association of Cerebrovascular Disease in Tohoku. Lateral and Medial Medullary Infarction: A Comparative Analysis of 214 Patients. Stroke, 2004: 35; 694-699.
10. Lee E, Kang DW, Kwon SU, Kim JS. Posterior Cerebral Artery Infarction: Diffusion-Weighted MRI Analysis of 205 Patients. Cerebrovasc Dis, 2009: 28; 298-305.
11. Canaple S, Bogousslavsky J. Multiple Large and Small Cerebellar Infarcts. J Neurol Neurosurg Psychiatry, 1999: 66; 739-745.
12. Kang DW, Lee SH, Bae HJ, Han MH, Yoon BW, Roh JK. Acute Bilateral Cerebellar Infarcts in the Territory of Posterior Inferior Cerebellar Artery. Neurology, 2000: 55; 582-584.
13. Donders RC; Dutch TMB Study Group. Clinical Features of Transient Monocular Blindness and the Likelihood of Atherosclerotic Lesions of the Internal Carotid Artery. J Neurol Neurosurg Psychiatry, 2001: 71; 247-249.
14. Jeffree RL, Stoodley MA. STA-MCA Bypass for Symptomatic Carotid Occlusion and Haemodynamic Impairment. J Clin Neurosci, 2009: 16; 226-235.
15. Chung WY, Sohn DW, Kim YJ, Oh S, Chai IH, Park YB, Choi YS. Absence of Postprandial Surge in Coronary Blood Flow Distal to Significant Stenosis: A Possible Mechanism of Postprandial Angina. J Am Coll Cardiol, 2002: 40; 1976-1983.

16. Aydogdu I, Ertekin C, Tarlaci S, Turman B, Kiylioglu N, Secil Y. Dysphagia in Lateral Medullary Infarction (Wallenberg's Syndrome): An Acute Disconnection Syndrome in Premotor Neurons Related to Swallowing Activity? Stroke, 2001: 32; 2081-2087.

17. Brandt T, Dieterich M. Vestibular Syndromes in the Roll Plane: Topographic Diagnosis from Brainstem to Cortex. Ann Neurol, 1994: 36; 337-347.

18. Elliott D. Migraine and Stroke: Current Perspectives. Neurol Res, 2008: 30; 801-812.

19. Serena J, Segura T, Perez-Ayuso MJ, Bassaganyas J, Molins A, Dávalos A. The Need to Quantify Right-to-Left Shunt in Acute Ischemic Stroke: A Case-Control Study. Stroke, 1998: 29; 1322-1328.

20. Konishi J, Yamada K, Kizu O, Ito H, Sugimura K, Yoshikawa K, Nakagawa M, Nishimura T. MR Tractography for the Evaluation of Functional Recovery from Lenticulostriate Infarcts. Neurology, 2005: 64; 108-113.

21. Carrera E, Bogousslavsky J. The Thalamus and Behavior: Effects of Anatomically Distinct Strokes. Neurology, 2006: 66; 1817-1823.

22. Ali S, Khan MA, Khealani B. Limb-Shaking Transient Ischemic Attacks: Case Report and Review of Literature. BMC Neurol, 2006: 5; 6.

23. Young RS, Zalneraitis EL. Marantic Endocarditis in Children and Young Adults: Clinical and Pathological Findings. Stroke, 1981: 12; 635-639.

24. Weingarten K, Filippi C, Barbut D, Zimmerman RD. The Neuroimaging Features of the Cardiolipin Antibody Syndrome. Clin Imaging, 1997: 6-12; 21.

25. Kimura K, Minematsu K, Nakajima M. Isolated Pulmonary Arteriovenous Fistula without Rendu-Osler-Weber Disease as a Cause of Cryptogenic Stroke. J Neurol Neurosurg Psychiatry, 2004: 75; 311-313.

26. Likosky DS, Marrin CA, Caplan LR, Baribeau YR, Morton JR, Weintraub RM, Hartman GS, Hernandez F Jr, Braff SP, Charlesworth DC, Malenka DJ, Ross CS, O'Connor GT; Northern New England Cardiovascular Disease Study Group. Determination of Etiologic Mechanisms of Strokes Secondary to Coronary Artery Bypass Graft Surgery. Stroke, 2003: 34; 2830-2834.

27. Stam J, De Bruijn SF, DeVeber G. Anticoagulation for Cerebral Sinus Thrombosis. Cochrane Database Syst Rev, 2002: (4); CD002005.

28. Dichgans M, Mayer M, Uttner I, Brüning R, Müller-Höcker J, Rungger G, Ebke M, Klockgether T, Gasser T. The Phenotypic Spectrum of CADASIL: Clinical Findings in 102 Cases. Ann Neurol, 1998: 44; 731-739.

29. O'Sullivan M, Jarosz JM, Martin RJ, Deasy N, Powell JF, Markus HS. MRI Hyperintensities of the Temporal Lobe and External Capsule in Patients with CADASIL. Neurology, 2001: 56; 628-634.

30. Iizuka T, Sakai F. Pathogenesis of Stroke-Like Episodes in MELAS: Analysis of Neurovascular Cellular Mechanisms. Curr Neurovasc Res, 2005: 2; 29-45.

31. Given CA 2nd, Huang-Hellinger F, Baker MD, Chepuri NB, Morris PP. Congenital Absence of the Internal

Carotid Artery: Case Reports and Review of the Collateral Circulation. AJNR Am J Neuroradiol, 2001 Nov.-Dec.: 22(10); 1953-1959.

32. Schwammenthal Y, Tanne D. Homocysteine, B-Vitamin Supplementation, and Stroke Prevention: From Observational to Interventional Trials. Lancet Neurol, 2004: 3; 493-495.

33. Marchal G, Young AR, Baron JC. Early Postischemic Hyperperfusion: Pathophysiologic Insights from Positron Emission Tomography. J Cereb Blood Flow Metab, 1999: 19; 467-482.

34. Pico F, Labreuche J, Touboul PJ, Amarenco P; GENIC Investigators. Intracranial Arterial Dolichoectasia and Its Relation with Atherosclerosis and Stroke Subtype. Neurology, 2003: 61; 1736-1742.

35. Koh MG, Phan TG, Atkinson KL, Wijdicks EF. Neuroimaging in Deteriorating Patients with Cerebellar Infarcts and Mass Effect. Stroke, 2000: 31; 2062-2067.

36. Mlekusch W, Schillinger M, Sabeti S, Nachtmann T, Lang W, Ahmadi R, Minar E. Hypotension and Bradycardia after Elective Carotid Stenting: Frequency and Risk Factors. J Endovasc Ther, 2003: 10; 851-859; Discussion 860-861.

37. Jung KH, Park SH, Chang GY. Imitative Arm Levitation from a Recurrent Right Thalamic Hemorrhage: A Case Report. Neurology, 2003: 61; 718.

38. Eidelberg D, Dhawan V, Moeller JR, et al. The Metabolic Landscape of Cortico-Basal Ganglionic Degeneration: Regional Asymmetries Studied with PET. J Neurol Neurosurg Psychiatry 1991: 54; 856-862.

39. Wieloch T, Nikolich K. Mechanisms of Neural Plasticity Following Brain Injury. Curr Opin Neurobiol, 2006: 16; 258-264.

40. Calautti C, Baron JC. Functional Neuroimaging Studies of Motor Recovery after Stroke in Adults: A Review. Stroke, 2003: 34; 1553-1566.